Welcome to
Ready Steady Baby!

Written by parents and healthcare professionals, this book is packed with useful information to take you all the way from the early stages of pregnancy to your baby's first birthday.

We've split the book into four sections which cover your pregnancy, giving birth, early days at home with your baby and your baby's development over the first year. Each section contains plenty of helpful advice from the experts (mums and midwives!) as well as at-a-glance summaries, letters and step-by-step guidance on everything from breastfeeding to nappy changing.

Throughout the book, we've referred to your baby as 'she'. We felt it made easier reading than saying 'he or she' throughout. So whether you have a 'he or she' – we hope you enjoy this book, your pregnancy and the newest member of your family when 'he or she' arrives!

Contents

you and your pregnancy

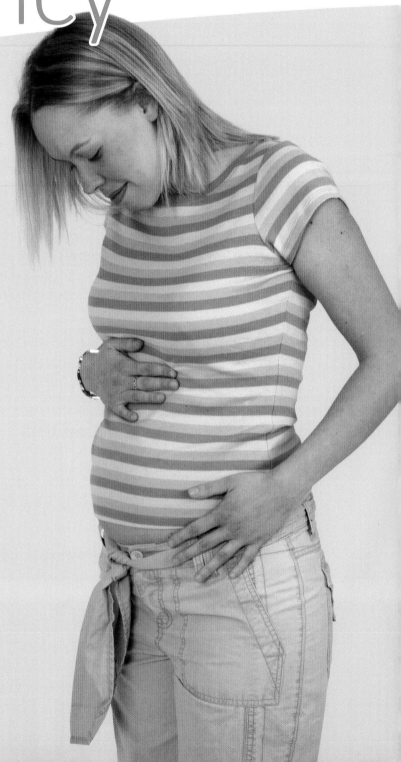

Section 1

Early pregnancy

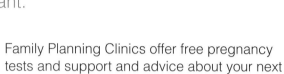

You've probably been given this book at your first appointment with your midwife, so chances are you already know that you're pregnant.

The first signs

The first sign of pregnancy tends to be missing a period, probably around two weeks after you've conceived. But this isn't foolproof. If your menstrual cycle isn't regular, you may not notice that you've missed a period. And some women have a bit of bleeding around the time they would have expected a period – caused by the embryo implanting itself in the womb lining – which can be confusing.

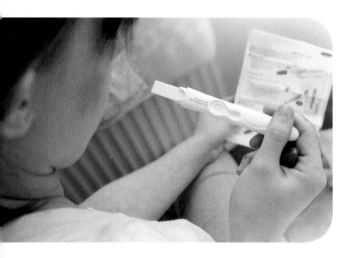

Home pregnancy tests are about 97% reliable. If you want, you can do one the first day you should have had a period. The test measures the amount of a hormone called human chorionic gonadotrophin (hCG) in your urine. This is the hormone that indicates you are pregnant. It is produced once the embryo is implanted and, in order for a positive pregnancy test, there must be sufficient levels for it to be detected. This is generally two weeks after conception (i.e. after the sperm has fertilised the egg, which in turn may be up to 24 hours after ovulation occurred).

Family Planning Clinics offer free pregnancy tests and support and advice about your next steps (see **Further help**, page 202).

If you think you may be pregnant and your period is late, phone your GP practice and arrange to visit a midwife to have it confirmed and to discuss what happens next.

Other signs of early pregnancy

Even before you miss a period, you may notice changes caused by pregnancy, especially if you're looking for signs. The changes are caused by hormones that can affect different parts of your body and the way you feel.

These are some of the signs:

- **Tender breasts:** your breasts may feel heavy and tender as they begin to make tissue for producing and storing milk.

- **Tiredness:** some women feel more exhausted in early pregnancy than at any other time.

- **Sickness:** feeling sick can happen very early on in pregnancy, but usually after the first four weeks. It can hit at any time of the day and not just in the morning. You may also go off some foods.

- **Going to the toilet more often:** you may find you feel as if you need to pass urine a lot more than usual.

- **Feeling emotional:** even if you really want to be pregnant, realising you are can come as a shock – not helped by all those hormones rushing around. Expect to feel a bit 'up and down'.

weeks 1-4

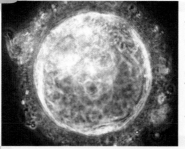

By the end of the first week after conception, the fertilised egg, called a blastocyst, has made its way along the fallopian tube and attached itself to the womb lining.

The outer cells of the embryo start to link into your blood supply so that they can start getting nourishment from it. This link will develop into the placenta, which is attached to the baby by a cord.

When the blastocyst is well implanted in the lining of the womb, it is called the embryo and is about the same size as the full stop at the end of this sentence.

The sex of your baby and all sorts of other things such as hair colour have already been decided – in fact, they were genetically determined from the moment of conception.

Your baby is growing at a faster rate than at any time in pregnancy but is still difficult to see without a magnifying glass.

How you may be feeling

Pregnancy hormones can really affect how you are feeling. Sometimes you can feel over the moon then down in the dumps within a matter of minutes. That's normal. It's also natural for you to have a few worries about your health and the health of your baby. You may be looking ahead to the birth and worrying about that. If you're on your own, you may be wondering how you'll manage (see **Being a single parent**, page 22). If something is really bothering you, talk to your midwife or GP about it – nobody is going to think you're being daft or wasting their time.

If you have a partner, he may also be worried about these things, as well as what's expected of him at the birth. Talking to each other about how you're feeling can help.

at a glance

✳ Hormones released by pregnancy can make you feel emotional.

✳ It's normal to feel worried, scared and excited and your midwife will understand.

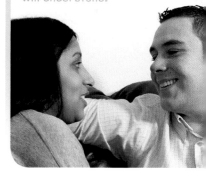

Q When is my baby due?

A. The start of your pregnancy is dated from the first day of your last actual period, although you probably conceived about a fortnight after this. That means that by the time you miss a period you are technically four weeks pregnant, based on the average menstrual cycle of 28 days. Pregnancy normally lasts between 38 and 42 weeks.

You'll be given a 'due date', but this is just a guideline. Most babies come in the fortnight before or after the due date. If you can't remember the date of your last period, other signs and symptoms can help your midwife or GP to tell how long you've been pregnant and you'll be offered an ultrasound scan (see **Having an ultrasound scan**, page 32).

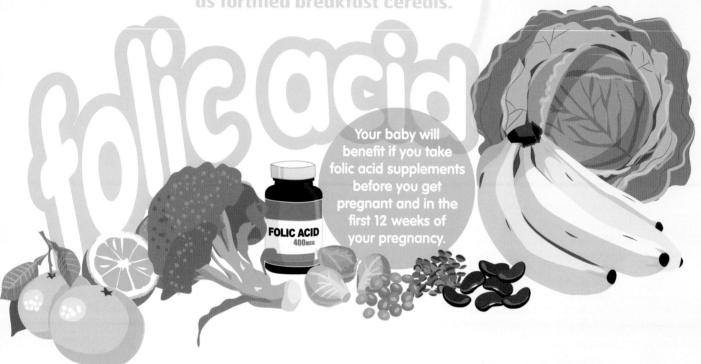

Folic acid is one of the B vitamins. It's found naturally in many foods and added to some manufactured foods such as fortified breakfast cereals.

folic acid

Your baby will benefit if you take folic acid supplements before you get pregnant and in the first 12 weeks of your pregnancy.

FOLIC ACID
400 MCG

Why is it important?

Folic acid helps babies develop. It helps prevent what are called neural tube defects, such as spina bifida, which are a cause of disability *(see page 40 for more information on neural tube defects)*. If you are pregnant, planning to get pregnant or there is a chance you might become pregnant, you should take a supplement and eat more foods containing folate (the natural form of folic acid).

With Healthy Start you get free vouchers for some food and vitamins. Ask your midwife if you qualify.

When should I take it and how much do I need to take?

Your baby's spine starts to grow very early in pregnancy – often before you even know you are expecting. This means it's important to make sure you're getting enough folic acid if you're hoping to get pregnant.

Currently it's recommended that you take a 400 mcg (0.4 mg) folic acid tablet every day before you get pregnant and for the first 12 weeks of pregnancy. You should also eat foods rich in folate *(see opposite)*. Speak to your GP if you have had a previous pregnancy with a neural tube problem, are on medication for epilepsy or have diabetes as you may need a higher dose.

How do I get it?

You can buy folic acid supplements from chemists, supermarkets or health food shops, or your GP can prescribe them if you get free prescriptions.

You can also eat foods containing folate, such as:

- green vegetables, particularly dark, leafy ones such as kale, broccoli and Brussels sprouts – steam rather than boil and be careful not to overcook as you will destroy some of the vitamins

- fortified breakfast cereals – some have extra folic acid added so check the label

- oranges, grapefruit, bananas, parsnips, black-eyed peas and pulses are also good sources of folate.

Vitamins and minerals while you are pregnant

A balanced and healthy diet is important if you are pregnant or trying to become pregnant. Although most vitamins and minerals are found in the foods you eat it is important to make sure you are getting enough iron and vitamin D. Your body needs time to build up iron throughout your pregnancy.

Iron

Pregnant women can have low levels of iron so it's important to make sure you have plenty of iron-rich foods such as meat, eggs, pulses, wholegrain bread and dark green vegetables. It's good to build up your iron levels throughout pregnancy and it's important to maintain them after your baby is born. The best way for your body to absorb iron is from the foods you eat.

Vitamin D

Vitamin D is needed to keep bones and teeth healthy. It's particularly important in preventing newborn babies from getting rickets. You should take supplements containing 10 mcg of vitamin D every day. Vitamin D is found in a few foods such as oily fish, eggs, margarine and fortified breakfast cereals but we get most of it from being outdoors and in the sun (though that is not an excuse to get sunburnt!). However, it is not possible to get enough vitamin D from food alone, and in Scotland there is not enough sunlight from November to April, so you should take vitamin D throughout your pregnancy and while you are breastfeeding. If you have dark skin, or cover your skin, you are particularly susceptible to vitamin D deficiency and should speak to your midwife or GP to get a suitable supplement.

at a glance

✳ You should take folic acid before you are pregnant and during your first 12 weeks of pregnancy.

✳ If you are eligible for Healthy Start (see page 64) you are entitled to free vitamins.

✳ Ask your midwife where to get vitamins while you are pregnant.

important note about vitamin A

Make sure you don't have too much vitamin A. This means you should avoid eating liver and liver products, such as pâté, and avoid taking supplements containing vitamin A or fish liver oils (which contain high levels of vitamin A).

You need some vitamin A, but having too much means that levels could build up and may harm your unborn baby. Ask your midwife or GP if you want more information (see **What foods to avoid**, pages 20–21).

Keeping fit and healthy during your pregnancy

Becoming pregnant can be a trigger for women and their partners to take steps to improve their health. It can be hard to make some healthy choices but the benefits for you and your baby are huge.

Research suggests that physical activity can have positive effects on your mood, self-esteem and body image. It can also help with sleep, stress, depression and anxiety.

Physical activity

Gentle physical activity is good for you, is usually safe and doesn't harm your baby's growth and development. Carrying on with your usual exercise routine is normally OK – unless you're into extreme sports – but check with your midwife and tell your instructor. Good activities include swimming and brisk walking, which are gentle in movement and intensity.

Stand tall!

You can strengthen your back and avoid backache by learning to 'stand tall'. Stand with your feet apart and let the weight of your body sink through to your feet. Imagine a string from the top of your head drawing you up towards the ceiling. Feel your spine lengthening.

When you stand, remember this posture. It helps to stop you slumping and sagging into your tummy.

Try not to sit for long periods of time. When sitting, tuck a small cushion into the small of your back to help you to sit up straight and comfortably. This takes the strain away from your back.

Yoga

Yoga is generally a safe and helpful form of exercise during pregnancy. The poses gently stretch the body and the breathing methods and emphasis on relaxation encourage peace and calm.

If you belong to a class, tell the teacher you are pregnant. If you want to start yoga, find a class specifically for pregnant women. Local authority education classes usually include yoga.

Low-impact aerobics

Aerobic exercise strengthens your heart and lungs and helps maintain muscle tone. Choose a class especially designed for expectant mothers, you'll enjoy the company of other women and be assured that the instructor is qualified to adapt the class especially for pregnancy. As long as you choose exercises which are low impact – meaning no high kicks and leaps, with one foot on the ground at all times to minimise stress on the joints – you should be able to continue your routine throughout your pregnancy, gradually tapering off towards the end.

Ask your midwife for a copy of NHS Health Scotland's, *Keeping active during and after pregnancy.*

Remaining active during your pregnancy has lots of benefits for you and will not harm your baby. This leaflet can also help you get started with gentle physical activity if you are not used to exercising.

Sports to avoid

Sports with a high potential for hard falls or ones where you might be thrown off-balance are not a good idea for pregnant women. These include horse-riding, downhill skiing, gymnastics and waterskiing. Additionally, most GPs and midwives recommend giving up cycling after six months, even if you're an experienced cyclist, because of the potential for falls. You can, however, use an exercise bike for as long as you like. If you are already active and have any concerns just check with your midwife whether it is safe to continue.

Swimming

Even if you haven't done much exercise before your pregnancy, you'll find swimming is easy. The water supports your whole body, so there's almost no risk of injury, and you can tone and stretch all over.

O **Many pools run 'aquanatal' classes, where you learn movements and exercises designed for pregnancy. These should be run by a specially trained midwife, or an obstetric physiotherapist with a midwife present.**

O **In any class, you should be given the chance to warm up with some gentle limb stretches, followed by movements which work round the body, and then maybe a swim.**

Walk to the shops or to work – or if that's too far, get off the bus a stop earlier or park a bit further away.

Take the stairs instead of lifts or escalators.

Make a point of taking time every few hours to do something active, even if it's just walking round the block.

at a glance

✳ If you already do a fitness class, tell your instructor that you are pregnant.

✳ Aquanatal classes are just for pregnant women and should be led by a specialist. Your leisure centre or council swimming pool should be able to give you details.

reasons to stop smoking

You don't need to do it alone. Your midwife or GP can refer you to a local stop smoking service or you can call Smokeline on 0800 84 84 84.

Why stop?

Most people are aware that smoking during pregnancy is harmful to both mum and baby. You may not be aware of the specific risks. Research has shown that growth is affected in babies whose mothers smoke during their pregnancy. They may be born too early and weigh less than normal. A baby with low birthweight may pick up infections more easily, can have difficulty breathing during and after birth and may have health and wellbeing problems that last through childhood and beyond.

There is strong evidence that if you, or someone in your household, smokes it will affect your pregnancy and your baby's health. So there has never been a better time to stop.

If you stop smoking, you will reduce risks to your pregnancy such as miscarriage or stillbirth, and risks to your baby such as cot death, and chronic conditions including asthma.

Carbon monoxide is a poisonous chemical that is present in your body because of smoking. Some areas now offer carbon monoxide testing to all pregnant women to show them the risks and help support their attempts to quit.

Passive smoking

Passive smoking can affect babies still in the womb. If you breathe in second-hand smoke, the chemicals in the smoke can make their way to your unborn baby.

Babies who live with people who smoke (parents, brothers, sisters or family friends) are likely to be harmed by breathing in second-hand smoke. Smoking regularly near a baby is one of the causes of cot death (see **Reducing the risk of cot death**, page 145). Other carers should not smoke near your baby. Smoke travels quickly – if you live with smokers who cannot stop, or there are smokers in the house, try to get them to smoke outside.

Your midwife or GP can put you in touch with stop smoking services, some specifically for pregnant women, who will support you and help you to stop. Help and information about services is also available from **Smokeline** on **0800 84 84 84** or visit **www.canstopsmoking.com**

> ❛I'd wanted to quit smoking for ages and had tried a few times but failed. This time it was different, however, as I was doing it for our baby. It was still tough but Smokeline really helped.❜
> *Danny, Glasgow*

Resources to help you **stop**

Stopping smoking is good for you and your baby. Stopping before or during early pregnancy is best but it is good for you and for your baby to stop at any point. Stopping smoking is good for your partner's health too.

Aspire to stop smoking

This booklet highlights the health benefits of stopping smoking, presents essential facts about nicotine replacement therapy and points smokers to sources of help and support.

How to stop smoking and stay stopped

This booklet will help smokers to decide if they are ready to stop and how to go about it.

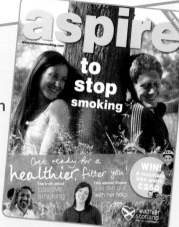

Fresh start

You'll find this booklet helpful if you're a smoker and you're trying for a baby, pregnant or have just had a baby. Find out about reasons to quit, the effects of smoking and how to get support when stopping smoking.

Passive Smoking – Unclouding the issue

This leaflet explains passive smoking and the associated health risks. You'll find answers to commonly asked questions and advice about reducing the harmful effects of passive smoking.

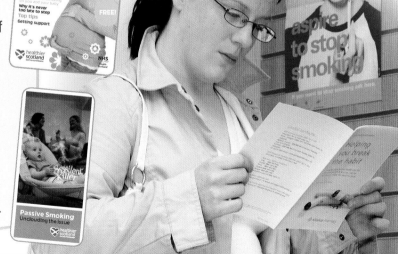

For help and information about stop smoking services visit www.canstopsmoking.com or call 0800 84 84 84.

Alcohol and your pregnancy

It is best to avoid alcohol completely during pregnancy, as any alcohol you drink while pregnant will reach your baby and may cause harm. Pregnant women and women trying to conceive should avoid drinking alcohol.

Fetal alcohol syndrome

There is evidence that even drinking one or two units per day can lead to health and development problems for your baby. Even small quantities of alcohol can cause fetal alcohol syndrome (FAS). FAS describes a range of effects on a baby's development as a result of her mother drinking too much during pregnancy.

There is no 'safe' time for drinking alcohol during your pregnancy and there is no 'safe' amount. We do know that the risk of damage increases the more you drink. Drinking no alcohol during your pregnancy is the best and safest choice.

While babies usually survive FAS, it can seriously harm their growth and mental development. Your midwife, GP or other healthcare staff will be happy to discuss any concerns you may have.

Breastfeeding and alcohol

Breastfeeding gives your baby the best possible start in life and it's unlikely that an occasional drink will harm either of you. We know that very small amounts of alcohol pass into your breast milk therefore it is best to keep your drinking to no more than one to two units once or twice a week.

If you regularly drink more than this amount it can affect your baby's development and reduce your milk supply. Small amounts of alcohol pass into breast milk, making it smell different, which may affect your baby's feeding, sleeping or digestion. If it's a special occasion and you know you are going to be having a drink, consider expressing your milk in advance *(see **Expressing your own milk**, page 125)*. To be on the safe side you may want to avoid alcohol altogether while you are breastfeeding.

Remember, if you are trying for a baby or are already pregnant, avoid alcohol altogether.

week 5

The embryo is still tiny – about the size of an apple pip – but is growing very quickly.

You may feel very tired.

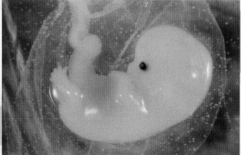

The heart and blood vessels are just beginning to form.

Your breasts may feel tender, as if you are starting your period.

Medicine and your pregnancy

Any drug may affect you or your baby, and that includes those you get on prescription, things you buy over the counter and some herbal remedies.

Prescribed drugs and over-the-counter medicines

You should tell your GP you're pregnant if you're being prescribed any medication, and also check with the pharmacist if it's OK to take it when you're pregnant. Check the label for yourself as well.

If you have a condition that means you take prescription drugs all the time, for example for epilepsy, talk to your GP or specialist when you are planning to get pregnant, or as soon as possible if the pregnancy was unplanned. You should not stop taking prescribed drugs without advice from your GP.

Illegal drugs

No recreational or street drugs are safe at any time and especially during pregnancy. Cocaine, crack, heroin, amphetamines and cannabis all affect your baby, directly or indirectly. Cocaine and crack are especially dangerous as they have an immediate effect on the baby's blood supply. The effect of Ecstasy on a baby's brain is not yet known. If you are addicted to drugs, help is available to support you. Some maternity units will provide special care or help if you need it. Your midwife, GP or antenatal clinic can put you in touch with specialist help. (See **Further help**, page 197).

If you feel that you cannot stop using any drug, help is available. Some maternity units have special addiction units. Being pregnant may be the extra encouragement you need to cope with giving up. Your midwife can put you in touch with support services, or speak to your GP.

eating well while you're pregnant

If you are eligible for Healthy Start you are entitled to vouchers for milk, fresh fruit and fresh vegetables. See page 64 or www.healthystart.nhs.uk for more information.

During pregnancy, making sure that your diet provides you with enough energy and nutrients for your baby to grow and develop is important. It is just as important to help keep you healthy and help your body to deal with all the changes taking place.

You are probably already wondering what you should and shouldn't be eating now that you are pregnant. The good news is that there is not much to avoid *(see pages 20 and 21 for more information)* and lots of things you enjoy already are good for you and your growing baby.

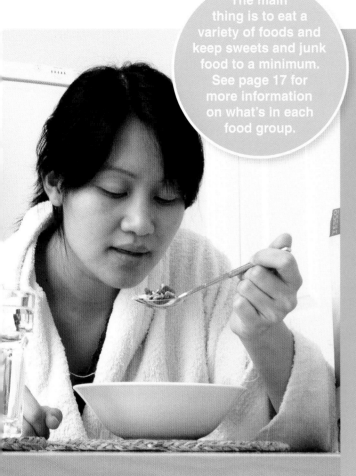

The main thing is to eat a variety of foods and keep sweets and junk food to a minimum. See page 17 for more information on what's in each food group.

What to **eat**

Eating a balanced and varied diet is the best way to be healthy and help your baby grow and develop. This means eating a range of things from the different food groups *(see page 17)* including:

○ lots of fruit and vegetables

○ plenty of starches like potatoes, pasta and wholegrain bread

○ protein-rich food including at least two portions of fish and one portion of oily fish a week

○ plenty of fibre which you'll find in fruit and vegetables as well as rice and wholegrain bread; eating fibre-rich foods will help you deal with constipation

○ dairy products like plain yoghurt, semi-skimmed milk and hard cheeses which will help you get enough calcium.

Healthy weight

Eating well will not only keep you and your baby healthy during your pregnancy but it is the best way to maintain a healthy weight throughout your pregnancy. A healthy diet can help you get back to your pre-pregnancy weight more quickly after the birth as well. Trying to lose weight while you are pregnant is not a good idea as it can harm both you and your baby. A diet made up of junk food and sweets will not do you much good. See page 54 for more information on weight gain in pregnancy.

Healthy drinks

It's essential to keep your fluid levels up by drinking plenty of water and fruit juices. Often we think we are hungry when in fact what we actually need is water.

Some experts suggest that the reason we retain water (and get puffy and bloated) is because we are not drinking enough of it. Drinking lots of water can also help with constipation.

Caffeine

If you are a regular coffee or tea drinker it's a good idea to try and cut back. High levels of caffeine can affect your baby's birthweight. For this reason it is important not to have more than 200 mg of caffeine a day. To give you an idea: an average cup of instant coffee has 75 mg of caffeine; regular brewed coffee has 100 mg; and regular tea has 50 mg. Cola and some 'energy drinks' also contain caffeine; 40 mg in a regular can of cola and as much as 80 mg in some energy drinks. You can substitute these with decaffeinated tea or coffee and look for drinks that are caffeine-free, such as herbal teas or fruit juices.

choosing
healthy foods

It can be more difficult to make healthy choices when eating take-aways or in restaurants. Sometimes it is hard to tell what is in your meal and how much you are going to be served; it's easy to end up eating much more salt and calories than you bargained for.

When going out to eat, or buying pre-cooked food, look for dishes that are steamed, grilled or poached rather than fried or battered. For example:

You're more likely to stick to a healthy diet if you enjoy what you eat!

○ grilled chicken or fish rather than a burger or fried fish
○ tomato or light vegetable sauces instead of heavy sauces or curries with lots of cream or cheese
○ lean meat, fish or pulses instead of pies, sausages or bacon

○ baked or boiled potatoes or plain rice rather than creamy potato dishes, chips or fried rice
○ fruit salad or sorbet instead of cakes, puddings or ice cream
○ wholegrain bread or toast instead of sweet pastries, muffins or croissants.

take it with you!
Snack **ideas:**

○ sandwiches or pitta bread filled with cottage cheese, chicken or lean ham
○ chopped vegetables such as carrot, cucumber or celery sticks
○ oat cakes, rice crackers or wholegrain biscuits with cheese such as cheddar or edam
○ low-fat cottage cheese or plain yoghurt

○ all kinds of fruit; bananas, apples and oranges are easy to transport and eat on the go
○ bottle of water or pure fruit juice

Carrying a snack or two with you is a good way to eat healthily throughout the day.

Eating from the **food groups**

Aim to eat a variety of foods from each of the food groups every day. That doesn't mean forcing yourself to eat things you don't like; after all, you are more likely to stick to healthy eating if you like what you are eating. Some research shows that the types of food you eat while pregnant and breastfeeding will later be what your baby enjoys too!

fruits and vegetables

Aim for at least five portions a day. A portion is an apple, or a glass of fruit juice, or three heaped tablespoons of vegetables or a dessert bowl full of salad. Incidentally, potatoes don't count in this category, as they are a starchy food *(see below left)* and fruit juice only counts as one portion.

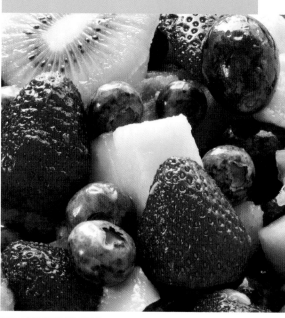

carbohydrates and starchy foods

These include breads, cereals, rice, potatoes and pasta and should be the main part of your diet. Try to eat at least three to four servings per day. Whole-meal or wholegrain starches are ideal as these types have more fibre and are more filling.

fats and sugars

Foods high in fat and sugar include cakes, biscuits, crisps, sugary drinks, sweets (including chocolate!) and anything fried in fat. Try to eat as little of this food group as possible.

dairy foods

Milk and other foods such as hard cheese *(see **What foods to avoid** on pages 20 and 21)* are a useful source of calcium. Calcium is very important in pregnancy because it helps your baby's developing bones to harden. Try to include a pint of skimmed or semi-skimmed milk per day in your diet or substitute a matchbox size piece of hard cheese, a carton of yoghurt or a milk pudding for one-third of a pint.

proteins

Lean meat, chicken, fish, eggs, pulses and nuts are all rich in protein and iron. Try to eat two portions a day. Pulses include peas and lentils, baked beans, runner beans, chickpeas, broadbeans, kidney beans and butter beans.

Tinned pulses are very quick and easy to use because they have already been soaked and cooked so only need to be heated or can be used cold. Try to avoid tins with added salt or sugar.

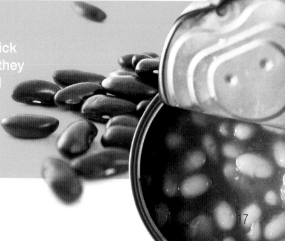

foods you can **eat safely**

Eggs – white and yolk – should be well cooked and not runny.

Healthy choices, such as eating well and stopping smoking, are good for you and your baby.

It can be confusing trying to work out which foods you can eat and which foods you should avoid when you are pregnant. Here are some foods you don't need to avoid:

○ shellfish, including prawns – as long as they are part of a hot meal and have been properly cooked

○ live or bio yoghurt

○ probiotic drinks

○ plain fromage frais

○ mayonnaise, ice cream, salad dressing, mousse – as long as they haven't been made using raw egg; if you're not sure about any of these foods when you are in a restaurant, ask staff for more information

○ creme fraiche

○ soured cream

○ spicy food

○ honey – is fine for pregnant women but is not suitable for babies under a year old

○ cheese – including hard cheese such as Cheddar and Parmesan; feta; ricotta; mascarpone; cream cheese; cottage cheese and processed cheese such as cheese spreads.

Q Can I eat peanuts when I'm pregnant? I'm not allergic to them but I'm worried about my baby.

A. If you would like to eat peanuts or foods containing peanuts (such as peanut butter) during pregnancy, you can choose to do so as part of a healthy balanced diet, unless you are allergic to them or a health professional advises you not to.

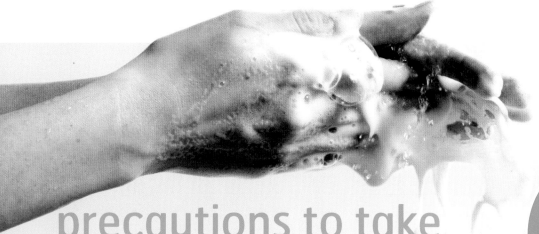

precautions to take when preparing food

Washing your hands before and during food preparation is one of the best ways to prevent the spread of bacteria.

○ Use the same care and attention to hygiene as you normally would.

○ Always wash your hands before and after handling food.

○ Wash all fruit and vegetables, including fruit or salad from pre-packed bags, before eating.

○ Always wash your hands (and any equipment used such as knives and cutting boards) after handling raw meat or fish.

○ Store raw foods separately from prepared foods. For example, raw meat should be kept in the lower part of the fridge.

○ Use separate chopping boards for meat and vegetables.

○ Ensure that precooked chilled ready meals are thoroughly heated and piping hot.

○ Make sure food is cooked through. Meats that aren't cooked can contain salmonella bacteria – be particularly careful with barbecues.

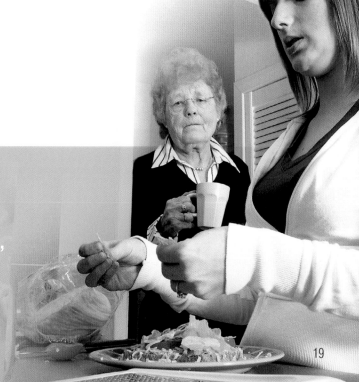

Always wear gloves for gardening or changing cat litter. This is to avoid toxoplasmosis, an infection caused by a parasite found in meat, cat faeces and soil, that is harmful to unborn babies. Wash your hands after handling or cleaning pets.

what foods to **avoid**

There are some foods you should avoid while you're pregnant.

Unpasteurised milk

This can contain a type of bacteria called listeria that can harm your baby. Pasteurised milk, which is what you get in most shops, is OK – in fact it is good for you and your baby.

Liver products and supplements containing vitamin A

Liver and liver products such as pâté or liver sausage may contain high levels of vitamin A which can be harmful to your baby. For the same reason, don't take vitamin A supplements. If you need extra supplements your GP will prescribe them.

Raw or partially cooked eggs

Don't eat raw eggs or food containing raw or partially cooked eggs, such as home-made mayonnaise (regular mayonnaise in jars is OK) puddings such as tiramisu and uncooked cheesecake. You should eat eggs cooked enough for both the white and yolk to be solid. This is to avoid the risk of salmonella, which causes food poisoning.

Some types of cheese

Avoid cheeses such as Camembert, Brie or chèvre (a type of goat's cheese), or others that have a similar rind. You should also avoid blue cheeses. These cheeses are made with mould and they can contain listeria, a type of bacteria that could harm your baby.

Pâté

Avoid all types of pâté, including vegetable. This is because pâté can contain listeria.

Raw or undercooked meats

Make sure you only eat meat that has been well cooked. This is especially important with poultry and products made from minced meat such as sausages and burgers. Make sure these are cooked until they are piping hot all the way through and no pink meat is left.

Always wash your hands after handling raw meat, and keep it separate from foods that are ready to eat. This is because raw meat contains bacteria that can cause food poisoning.

Some foods are risky while you are pregnant either because they could harm your baby or because they may make you ill. Visit www.eatwell.gov.uk

Some types of fish

You can eat most types of fish when pregnant, but there are a few to either avoid or limit the amount you eat.

Avoid eating any shark, swordfish and marlin.

Have no more than two portions of oily fish a week. Oily fish includes fresh tuna (tinned tuna does not count as oily fish), mackerel, herring, sardines and trout.

Limit the amount of fresh tuna you eat in a week to no more than two tuna steaks (weighing about 140 g cooked or 170 g raw) or four medium sized tins of tuna (with a drained weight of about 140 g per can). This is because of the levels of mercury which can harm a baby's developing nervous system.

Raw shellfish

Avoid raw shellfish when you are pregnant because it can contain harmful bacteria and viruses that can cause food poisoning. It's OK to eat shellfish, including prawns, if they have been properly cooked.

Alcohol

It is recommended that you do not drink any alcohol during your pregnancy or when trying for a baby. For more information on alcohol and pregnancy see page 12.

Undercooked ready meals

Avoid eating ready meals that are undercooked. Make sure that you heat them until they are piping hot all the way through.

You may have heard that some women have chosen not to eat peanuts when they are pregnant. The government had previously advised women to avoid eating peanuts if there was a history of allergy in the child's immediate family. However, this advice has now been changed because there is no clear evidence to support this. For general information on food allergy, including peanut allergy, visit: www.eatwell.gov.uk/healthissues/foodintolerance/foodintolerancetypes/

week 6

There are three layers in the embryo now. The first will become the nervous system and brain, the second will be the major organs such as the digestive system and lungs, and the third will be the heart, blood system, muscles and skeleton.

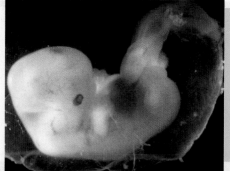

If you haven't already started to feel sick, this could be the week you do, although some women go through pregnancy without feeling sick at all.

The embryo is starting to look like a little tadpole but the 'tail bone' will disappear and become the coccyx.

Pregnancy hormones are kicking in and you may be very emotional.

If you haven't already been taking a folic acid supplement, you should start taking it now to prevent your baby from getting neural tube defects. Keep taking it until you are 12 weeks pregnant.

At this point, the embryo is the size of the nail on your little finger.

Being a single parent

If you're on your own, the whole business of pregnancy can seem daunting. You may feel lonely, especially if it seems as though everyone else has a partner to help them through it.

You're not alone – there's extra help available. Don't be afraid to ask.

Ask for support and help

You may be worried about going through the birth on your own and how you'll cope when the baby is born and is growing up.

You may have family or friends nearby and they'll probably be happy to help out if you let them know what you need. That may be anything from a shoulder to cry on (everyone gets weepy during pregnancy) to going along to antenatal classes with you. You may also want to think about who you'd like with you at the birth. Your mum? Your best pal? Both?

It may help to talk to someone who is in the same situation or who has been through it.

Your midwife may be able to put you in touch with someone or there are national helplines *(see **Further help**, page 205)* such as the One Parent Families Scotland helpline on **0808 801 0323.** You can also get a copy of their *Young Mum's Guide* or *Top Ten Tips for Lone Parents* by calling the helpline.

The thought of being a single mother can be pretty scary, but there are people to help you through it.

As for after your baby is born – well, yes, it is tougher to bring up a child by yourself. But the most important thing that every baby and child needs is someone to love her and care for her. You can do that.

week

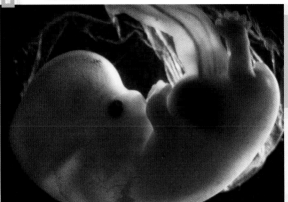

Your baby's heart is already beating and her lungs have just started to form.

Foods may taste different and your likes and dislikes may change.

Your baby may start to move around now but you won't feel any movement for a while yet.

Your baby has tiny hands and feet with webbed fingers and toes.

How will you feed your baby?

How you will feed your baby is an important decision which can have lifelong benefits for your health as well as your baby's.

Making the right choice

Breastfeeding is the healthiest option for you and your baby. If you choose not to breastfeed, formula substitutes are available. Whatever you decide, it's important that you are prepared and feel confident about how to feed your baby.

Breastfeeding has many health benefits *(see pages 122–123)*. It's also convenient and some mums feel it helps them to bond with and get to know their baby.

Most Scottish maternity hospitals are taking part in the UNICEF UK Baby Friendly Award Scheme, which means that staff are trained to give you as much support as you need to breastfeed. It can also be a good idea to chat to a friend who successfully breastfed her baby.

Ask your midwife or health visitor for a copy of NHS Health Scotland's *Off to a good start* for detailed information on breastfeeding, and see also the breastfeeding section on pages 122–125. Some areas run breastfeeding workshops, so ask your midwife if there are any in your area.

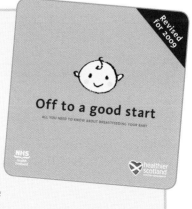

Off to a good start

ALL YOU NEED TO KNOW ABOUT BREASTFEEDING YOUR BABY

Revised for 2009

NHS
National Health Scotland

healthier scotland

If you would like to eat peanuts or foods containing peanuts (such as peanut butter) while breastfeeding, you can choose to do so as part of a healthy balanced diet, unless you are allergic to them or your health professional advises you not to.

Antenatal care: your healthcare during pregnancy

Antenatal care means the care you receive throughout your pregnancy and before birth. Antenatal care aims to ensure a healthy pregnancy for you and your developing baby.

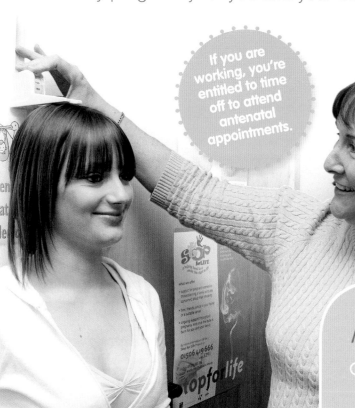

If you are working, you're entitled to time off to attend antenatal appointments.

Some women like to take along a list of questions so they don't forget anything, while others like to jot down notes to look at afterwards.

Pregnant – what next?

healthier scotland

NHS

What to expect

Your antenatal care aims to check that you and your baby are well, to pick up any problems before they become serious and to give you the chance to ask questions. Some may be at hospital but most will probably take place at the midwives' or GPs' clinic or at home *(see **Antenatal care: who's involved in looking after you?**, page 28).*

Antenatal care:

○ is the care you can expect to receive from your midwife and GP during your pregnancy, whether you plan to give birth at home or in hospital

○ includes between eight and **10** different appointments over the course of your pregnancy

○ will ask about aspects of your lifestyle that you may want to consider (such as diet, exercise, alcohol and drug intake, sexual activity and smoking)

○ will offer routine screening tests for specific conditions.

week 8

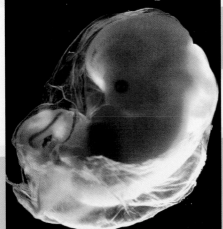

Your baby is about 1.6 cm (about half an inch) from the top of her head to her bottom. She is measured this way until around week 20 when the measurement includes the legs.

She's floating inside the amniotic sac (bag of waters) which will protect her throughout pregnancy.

Tiny buds are developing on the embryo that will become arms and legs.

Your hair may be getting thicker.

You may need to go to the toilet more because your uterus has doubled in size and is putting pressure on your bladder.

The booking appointment

This is your first major appointment and usually takes place when you're between eight and 12 weeks pregnant. You'll be seen by a midwife either at her clinic (which may be at your GP practice) or in your home. This visit can last around an hour and gives you a chance to talk to the midwife about the care you'll have during your pregnancy and after your baby is born.

What happens at your booking appointment

Don't expect to be in and out in five minutes! There's a lot to get through. These are some of the things that could happen:

- you'll be asked lots of questions about your health and family health

- the midwife will explain the different options for antenatal care in your area

- the midwife will check things including your weight, height and blood pressure

- you may have to give a urine sample or bring one with you

- the midwife will offer to take some blood for tests *(see **Tests and checks you may have during pregnancy**, page 36)* and you will get information about screening tests for you and your baby

- you may be asked where you want to have your baby but remember you don't have to make up your mind now; even if you do, you can change it later

- above all, this appointment is your chance to ask all the questions that you have been thinking about – such as how you feel about the pregnancy as well as the physical changes in your body

- you will get information about the benefits you are entitled to *(see page 62)*.

At a glance

✳ There are different types of antenatal care and what you are offered can depend on which part of the country you live in and whether you have special needs.

✳ Several different people may be involved in your care, including midwives, your GP and hospital doctors.

✳ Take your antenatal notes with you if you're away from home for any length of time.

Where will you give birth?

You'll usually be asked to 'book' where you want to give birth near the start of your pregnancy but you can change your mind later. It's important that your midwife knows what you want.

Choosing where to give birth

Depending where you live, you may have a choice where you can give birth. It also makes sense to ask around and find out what other people's experiences have been like. Some of the main options that may be available in your area are listed here.

At home

If you are thinking about a home birth you should discuss your care options with your midwife. For a home birth you will be offered support from your midwife and the Scottish Ambulance Service as well as support from a linked maternity unit. In some remote or rural areas in Scotland, it may not be feasible to have a home birth if you are too far from a hospital, in case you want an epidural or there are complications. In these circumstances, home birth is possible but may not be recommended. There is no evidence that a planned home birth is riskier than a hospital birth for women who are not expected to have problems with pregnancy or birth.

Community maternity unit

This may be available in your area, particularly in more rural parts of Scotland. In many cases, this unit will be led by midwives and it is suitable for women expected to have a normal pregnancy and birth. It will have links with a hospital maternity unit in case you need to be transferred.

Midwife-led unit in hospital

Some hospitals have midwife-led units where midwives are responsible for running the unit. Usually this is for women who are expecting a normal birth.

Consultant-led unit in hospital

This will normally be where you give birth if you expect to need care from a doctor. There may be more than one consultant-led unit in your area. Some women who don't expect to have problems prefer to give birth in these units, as they feel reassured by having specialist medical care close at hand. Midwives carry out most of the care in these units.

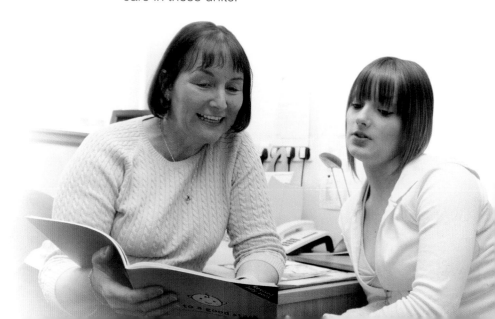

week 9

Your baby is about 2.5 cm (almost an inch) long from the top of her head to her bottom.

She has eyelids but they will stay closed for a few weeks yet.

The ends of her arms and legs are starting to look like hands and feet though they are not yet fully formed.

You don't look pregnant yet but your waistline may be starting to thicken and your breasts are probably getting larger – get measured for a new bra to ensure you're getting enough breast support.

at a glance

✳ You have the right to choose where you give birth.

✳ You can talk over your options with your midwife, partner, and other women in the area who have recently given birth.

✳ You should be given enough information to make an informed choice, balancing risks and taking into account what's available in your area.

It's not too soon to think about where and how you want to give birth.

your antenatal notes

Everything that happens during antenatal care is written in your notes. You should take them with you whenever you see your midwife or any other healthcare professional.

Your notes will have information including details of previous pregnancies and the results of any tests you have had.

Some women like to keep a copy of what they want to happen when they give birth (see **Planning for the birth**, *page 70*) with their notes.

Sometimes references in your notes will be abbreviated or contain medical jargon you may not understand. If you don't understand something, or have questions, ask your midwife who will be happy to explain. (See **Glossary** *for more information, pages 208–209).*

Antenatal care: who's involved in looking after you?

You'll perhaps have more to do with the NHS in the next few months than you will for the rest of your life – unless you have another baby, that is! For each pregnancy, there will be a 'lead professional' – usually the midwife – but it may be your GP or obstetrician. Here's a list of the people you may come across and what they do:

Health professionals may be male or female. You have the right to ask to be seen by female staff, but this may not always be possible. Interpreters (usually female) are provided if you need them.

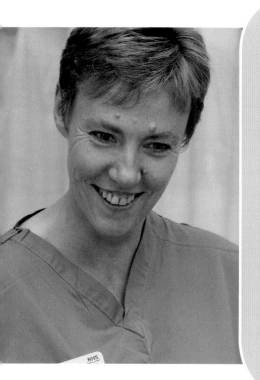

Midwife: the main provider of care for most pregnant women. Midwives are highly-skilled, qualified professionals who care for women during normal pregnancy, childbirth and after the birth. You will be introduced to your midwife, who will care for you during your pregnancy and when you go home. You may meet different members of a team of midwives throughout your pregnancy.

Midwives are trained to make sure everything goes as well as possible and to recognise any potential problems for you and your baby. Midwives work both in maternity units and in the community, often in a team system. The style of care may depend on where you live. Community midwives may visit you at home before the birth and will continue to care for you after the birth.

Obstetrician: a doctor who specialises in pregnancy and childbirth. You may see an obstetrician or another qualified doctor who is trained in obstetrics. Obstetricians are likely to be heavily involved if there is a problem with your pregnancy or birth but, if everything is OK, chances are you may not need to see one.

GP: general practitioners are qualified doctors; they may have an extra qualification in obstetrics. Your GP may provide your antenatal care.

week 10-11

Your baby's arms and legs are getting longer and her elbows can bend.

You'll probably be feeling hungrier than usual – your body is busy growing a baby after all!

All the activity going on inside you is probably making you very tired but you may find it hard to sleep.

Your baby's heart has developed fully and is working but still can't be heard by your midwife.

Her head looks big compared with the rest of the body, but don't worry, her body will catch up.

She's about 4 cm (about 1½ inches) long from head to bottom and weighs as much as a large grape.

Toes and fingers are beginning to lose their webbing and nails are forming.

Health visitor: also known as a public health nurse. A health visitor is a nurse who has had extra training in child development and health promotion and who works in the community, either with a specific GP practice (or practices) or within a specific area. Health visitors give support and advice to parents and their children until the age of five and have a role in protecting the health of the whole community. They have experience and knowledge about what's going on in your area. You can visit your health visitor at the baby clinic, or he or she may come to meet you for the first time while you are still pregnant. Your health visitor also makes home visits.

Paediatrician: a doctor who specialises in babies and children. A neonatologist is a paediatrician who specialises in newborn babies. If there are any worries about your baby's health, a paediatrician may be present at the birth. A paediatrician may also check your baby over before you go home from hospital, although this is increasingly being done by midwives who have completed training in this specialised area of care (see **Further help**, page 206).

Obstetric physiotherapist: the role of the obstetric physiotherapist is to help you cope with the changes in your body's shape and functions during pregnancy and after the birth.

Social worker: social workers can help to support families who have additional needs or are struggling to cope, if there are concerns for the welfare of the child, or if the child or a family member has a disability. Your midwife or GP can put you in touch with a social worker if necessary.

Dietician: dieticians can give advice on food and nutrition, particularly if you have specific needs, for example if you have diabetes.

Ultrasonographer: the professional who operates the ultrasound scanning equipment (see **Having an ultrasound scan**, page 32). This may be a midwife, a radiographer or an obstetrician.

Radiologist: a doctor who specialises in ultrasound.

Students and trainee health professionals: midwives, doctors and other health professionals need to be trained. You may be asked if you mind if students take part. You have the right to refuse.

Health professionals may ask you about your experience of care during your pregnancy, or ask you to complete a questionnaire. By doing this you provide information which is used to improve healthcare for pregnant women, mothers and babies. Any information you give is confidential and you don't have to answer questions.

When pregnancy goes wrong

Losing a baby, no matter where you are in your pregnancy, is a very difficult experience. Your midwife and your GP can reassure you that you are in no way to blame.

Miscarriage in early pregnancy

Most miscarriages happen in the first three months of pregnancy and in most cases there is no clear reason why it happens. Research shows it is very unlikely that anything a pregnant woman did or didn't do will have caused the miscarriage. Sadly, for most women, the cause is unexplained.

As many as one in five pregnancies can end in miscarriage. A miscarriage, also called a 'spontaneous abortion', means losing your baby (technically the fetus) before 24 weeks.

Symptoms of miscarriage

While some spotting of blood is quite common in early pregnancy, it's worth mentioning to your midwife. Heavier bleeding, possibly accompanied by cramps that feel like bad period pain, could be the start of a miscarriage. If this happens, you should call your midwife or GP immediately.

How you may be feeling

Even though miscarriage is common, that doesn't make it any less upsetting. Family and friends will try to cheer you up and they mean well but sometimes it doesn't help. You and your partner need to give yourself time to grieve. It can help to talk it over with others who have been through the same thing. Your midwife may be able to put you in touch with a local support group (see **Further help**, page 206).

If you experience a late miscarriage or a stillbirth you will need midwifery care to make sure your body is recovering.

domestic abuse and pregnancy

One in 10 women in Scotland experience domestic abuse each year (one in five at some point in their lives), and a third of all cases begin in pregnancy. Domestic abuse isn't just about violence. It can be sexual, emotional, psychological, or a combination of these.

Abuse when you are pregnant can affect your unborn child and cause complications in pregnancy.

You can talk to your midwife or GP or health visitor/public health nurse. The Scottish Domestic Abuse helpline, **0800 027 1234**, is a confidential service providing information and advice. The number won't show up on your phone bill.

The sooner you seek help the better, either through support or, if necessary, by seeking refuge.

Q *My partner has just had a miscarriage. She was eight weeks pregnant and we were both really looking forward to the baby. I'm trying to give her all the support I can but I find it hard to talk about it. It seems all the help that's available is aimed at her and I can't help feeling left out.*

A. It can be hard to talk to your partner about how you're feeling because you may think you'll just upset her more. But you're doing the right thing by trying to support her and realising that you need help yourself. Ask your midwife or GP for details of support groups in your area and think about whether there's someone else you may find it easier to talk to about how you're feeling.

Cervical incompetence

Occasionally, miscarriages are caused by a condition that is known as cervical incompetence. This means that the cervix or neck of the womb doesn't stay closed but starts to dilate (open). In these circumstances, the baby may be lost before the 20th week. If this has been a problem for you in the past, speak to your midwife or GP about getting extra help early in pregnancy to reduce the risk of it happening again.

Multiple miscarriages

Help is available for women who have had more than one miscarriage. Your GP can refer you to a specialist who can investigate possible causes. If you've had a miscarriage before, make sure your midwife or GP know so that you can get help to reduce the risks.

Other circumstances

Ectopic pregnancy

This means the pregnancy has developed outside the uterus, usually in the fallopian tube. You will need medical help as it is dangerous for you. Unfortunately an ectopic pregnancy can't be saved. It usually becomes apparent at about six weeks. Symptoms may include pain low down in the abdomen, bleeding, paleness and sweating. It's important to seek medical help quickly as early treatment means it is more likely that the fallopian tube can be saved and your fertility may not be affected.

Stillbirth

It's rare for a baby to die in the uterus or at birth – it happens in only one in 200 pregnancies. Like miscarriage, often we just don't know why it happens. Sometimes there simply isn't an explanation. It can help to talk to others in the same situation *(see **Further help**, page 204).*

at a glance

- As many as one in five pregnancies end in miscarriage.
- Most miscarriages occur in the first three months of pregnancy.
- Most women who have had a miscarriage go on to have a healthy pregnancy in the future.
- This is a difficult time for your partner too. It's important to support each other and ask for help and support from others if you need it.

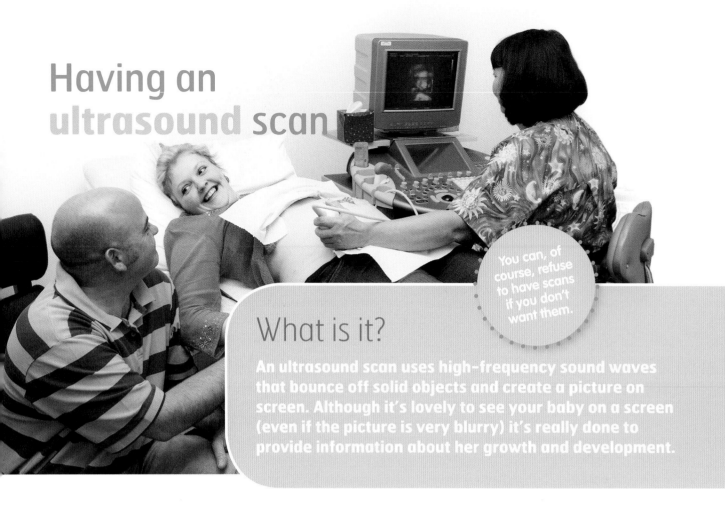

Having an ultrasound scan

You can, of course, refuse to have scans if you don't want them.

What is it?

An ultrasound scan uses high-frequency sound waves that bounce off solid objects and create a picture on screen. Although it's lovely to see your baby on a screen (even if the picture is very blurry) it's really done to provide information about her growth and development.

Things your ultrasound can show:

○ Your baby's size, which is important for dating the pregnancy and finding out when the baby is due.

○ The way your baby is lying in the uterus, which may be important at the end of your pregnancy.

○ Whether twins (or more!) are in there.

○ The development of your baby's organs and bones, including the spine. An ultrasound scan can also show some abnormalities or problems, but it is not always possible to identify them.

○ Where the placenta is lying. In late pregnancy, a low-lying placenta may cause bleeding and block your baby's way out, so you may need a Caesarean section *(see page 80)*.

Ultrasound can also be used to find out the exact position of the baby to allow the doctor to carry out other tests such as amniocentesis or chorionic villus sampling (CVS) *(see page 39)*.

In the few cases where ultrasound reveals an unexpected problem, you may be referred for further diagnostic tests.

National guidelines say that women should be offered two scans at around 12 and 20 weeks. The first is known as the 'dating scan' because it helps to show how many weeks pregnant you are. The second is a more detailed scan that helps to pick up any problems. In practice, you may find that provision varies across the country. In some areas you may be offered a special ultrasound called a 'nuchal translucency scan' (NT) which is done at 11 to 13 weeks, in combination with a blood test, as a screening test for Down's syndrome. Your midwife will give you information about what is available in your area.

week 12

Your baby is waving her legs and she can curl her fingers and toes but you won't feel this yet.

She has 20 little buds, which will eventually become teeth.

You may have an ultrasound now, although this varies.

Your waist may be getting a bit thicker and some women begin to develop a small bump at this stage.

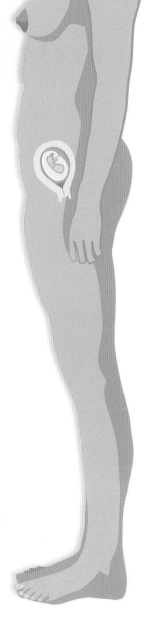

at a glance

✳ Ultrasound scans are a way to get information about your baby's growth and development.

✳ They are also the first chance to get a look at your baby!

✳ You should be offered two scans, at around 12 and 20 weeks, but in practice this varies around Scotland.

✳ If you don't want a scan your decision will be respected.

Points to remember:

○ Ask for a picture to take away with you. Some units make a charge or ask for a donation for this.

○ Ask about anything that is worrying you.

What actually happens?

Depending on how many weeks pregnant you are, you will probably have to fill your bladder before a scan by drinking lots of water. This means your bladder pushes the uterus up and lets the ultrasonographer get a better picture. It's a bit uncomfortable for you as you may want to go to the toilet, but it is painless.

How it's done

You lie down on a couch and the ultrasonographer stands or sits next to you. You'll need to adjust your clothes so that your abdomen (tummy) is uncovered. Cold gel is spread on your abdomen then a hand-held instrument (called a transducer) which looks a bit like a microphone is rolled over your abdomen. This picks up a picture of everything underneath it and transmits it to a screen.

When to tell people

Most people wait until the end of the first trimester (after 12 weeks) until they announce they're pregnant. That's the stage when there is much less risk of miscarriage, and you may well have had an ultrasound *(see page 32)* and even seen your baby on screen.

Who to tell

You may want to tell very close friends and family before 12 weeks, but it's really up to you and your partner and it should be a joint decision. There is no right or wrong time.

Bear in mind that some people will take this opportunity to pass on advice, including horror stories. While it can be good to hear about other people's experiences, don't feel you have to take their advice or feel bullied into making any choices which you're not happy with. It's your baby so it's up to you.

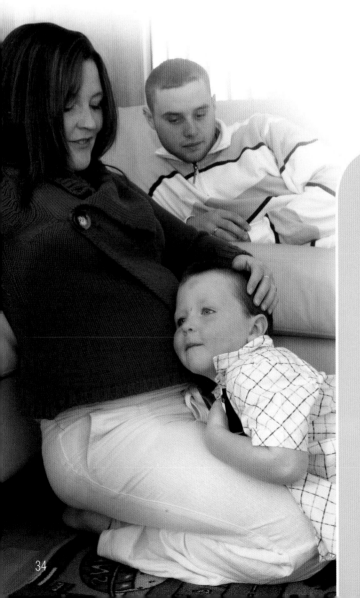

Telling children

Parents who already have a young child or children sometimes decide not to tell them until the pregnancy is further on. Nine months is a long time to a toddler! Children may well pick up on the information if other people know, however, so you need to judge for yourself how you want to handle it.

Telling children about pregnancy can raise lots of questions for them, and depending on their age, they may want to know how it happens! If you would like help or advice talking about this with your children ask your midwife.

week 13-14

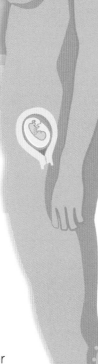

Your baby's ears have developed but she can't hear yet. The fetus looks like a tiny baby.

The liver, kidneys, digestive system and lungs are maturing.

You should not be feeling as sick as you were (although for some women sickness goes on longer).

Although birth is still many months away, your breasts may already be making colostrum – the fluid that will feed your baby for her first few days.

The placenta is now your baby's source of nourishment.

Your baby is about 7 cm (almost 3 inches) from her head to her bottom.

You may start to develop a dark line from your tummy button (navel) to your pubic hair. This is called the 'linea nigra'.

at a glance

※ Some people want to tell everyone straight away – others don't.

※ Some women like to wait until they are 13 weeks pregnant, when they are much less likely to have a miscarriage.

※ If you are working, you have to tell your employer by the 15th week before the baby is due.

The best time to take a holiday or longer trip is between 13 and 26 weeks (the second trimester).

Telling work

What you decide to tell colleagues and employers, and when, will depend on a few things, including your relationship with your boss and how you are feeling early in pregnancy. It's a good idea to make sure your employer hears the news from you, not through workplace gossip. You may not want to tell anyone until you're past the first trimester, but you may need to let people know sooner if, for example, you're suffering bad morning sickness, are particularly tired or are having other health problems.

Your antenatal rights don't kick in until you've notified your employer. You have to tell your employer by the 15th week before the baby is due (see **Maternity Leave and other payments and benefits**, page 62).

Tests and checks you may have during pregnancy

Always ask the reason for tests – they may be routine and straightforward to the health professionals carrying them out, but not to you.

Routine tests

You will be offered several tests and checks as an important part of your care during pregnancy. These tests are intended to help protect you and your baby's health.

It's up to you whether you have the tests. The test results are confidential and only you and the healthcare professionals closely involved with your care will be told the results. Nobody else will be told the results without your permission. Your midwife will be happy to discuss tests currently offered in your area with you.

Routine blood tests

You will be offered at least one blood test in pregnancy, usually taken at your first antenatal appointment, although different regions in Scotland may do this at different times. A blood test just means taking a little blood from a vein in your arm. The blood is drawn up into a syringe or vacuum tube. A blood test shouldn't be painful but may be uncomfortable, and there may be slight bruising for a day or so afterwards.

It is your decision whether to accept these tests or not, and it won't affect the quality of your care. However, having the tests could help you make decisions about the care of your baby, both before and after birth. All results are confidential and only health professionals closely involved in your care will be able to see them. No one will be told about your results without your consent.

Blood tests can include:

- **Full blood count:** the full blood count (FBC) is a good all-round measure of health. If it is low it indicates you could be anaemic.

- **Blood group:** this identifies your blood group (A, B, O or AB). It can also identify whether there are any blood group antibodies in your blood.

- **Rhesus positive or negative:** if you are rhesus positive, no further action will be taken. If you are rhesus negative, you will be offered injections called anti-D, which help prevent a serious illness for any future babies you may have. One in six women are rhesus negative.

- **Rubella (German measles):** rubella is usually a mild illness, but if you are infected in the first 20 weeks of pregnancy it can harm your baby and may affect development, causing deafness and blindness for example. This test, unlike the others, is to make sure you are already protected. You may have been immunised in childhood, but if you are not immune or have low levels of immunity, you will be given health advice and offered immunisation after the birth. You should contact your midwife or GP if you develop a rash or come into contact with someone with a rash during pregnancy.

- **Syphilis:** this is a sexually acquired infection. It is rare but, if undetected, it can seriously damage your health and that of your baby by causing developmental difficulties. Effective treatment (a course of antibiotics) is available.

- **Hepatitis B:** this is a viral infection which causes liver disease and can be passed from mother to baby during or just after delivery. If you test positive, your baby will receive a complete course of a very effective vaccine and possibly injections of antibodies called immunoglobulin immediately after the birth.

- **HIV:** the Human Immunodeficiency Virus (HIV) is the virus that causes Acquired Immunodeficiency Syndrome (AIDS). Infected pregnant women can pass HIV to their babies during pregnancy, childbirth and also through breastfeeding. HIV attacks the body's immune system and destroys the body's defences to infection. It can take years for HIV to do enough damage for you to become ill, so usually the only way to tell if you are infected is to take a test. If your HIV result is positive, advice and treatment under the guidance of specialists will be offered.

Interventions include treatment with special drugs and advice about the best type of delivery and the best method of feeding your baby to reduce the risk of her also getting the infection. For more information about HIV and AIDS, *(see **Further help**, pages 203–204).*

Test results

You will be told when you can expect your results at the time they are arranged. If there is a problem or anything you should know, you will be contacted as quickly as possible. If you have any questions or concerns about these tests, please ask at your next clinic visit or contact your midwife.

You can decide at any point that you do not want to be tested or you can choose to have only some of the tests offered to you.

You will receive further information on screening tests offered during pregnancy from your midwife and they will be happy to answer any questions.

Routine checks

Blood pressure

Your blood pressure is checked at most appointments. It is normally taken in early pregnancy to get a baseline and later to make sure you have no signs of pre-eclampsia or pregnancy-induced hypertension *(see page 79)*. The midwife wraps a fabric band around your arm and inflates it with a small pump. The band is linked to a blood pressure measure. As it deflates, the midwife uses a stethoscope to listen to changes in your pulse.

A high reading may give cause for concern – the test may be done again, 10 or 20 minutes later, to make doubly sure.

Urine

Your urine will be tested for protein and sugar. A special strip is dipped into a sample which you either bring with you or produce at the appointment. Some women develop a particular sort of diabetes that occurs in pregnancy – gestational diabetes. This may show as sugar in the urine. Protein may indicate pre-eclampsia. Infections of the kidney and bladder may show up here too.

Abdomen

Your abdomen (tummy) will be examined at each visit. This means the midwife feels the way your baby is lying, and her size and the height of your uterus, by moving her hands around the outside of your abdomen.

> I decided to have further tests although I knew I would go ahead with the pregnancy whatever the results. My partner and I wanted to have time to prepare if we were going to have a child with a disability.
> *Joanne, Aberdeen*

Screening and diagnostic tests for spina bifida and Down's syndrome

Most babies are born perfectly healthy, but a few are born with conditions such as spina bifida, Down's syndrome or other chromosomal abnormalities *(see page 40)*. There are tests available during pregnancy that can help to detect these rare conditions.

You can choose whether or not to have these tests, and you may want to discuss this with your midwife. In most cases further tests show your baby is healthy. If not, you will be offered counselling to help you decide what to do.

There are two types of test: screening, which is offered to everyone and is intended to show whether there is a low chance or a high chance of your baby having a condition such as Down's syndrome; and diagnostic, which means further tests which may be offered to confirm a condition depending on the results of the screening test. About 1 in 10 women will be offered second follow-up tests such as amniocentesis or ultrasound. While screening offers a good way to assess how likely it is that your baby has one of these conditions, it is not perfect and will not detect all problems.

Screening test

The screening test involves taking a blood sample from your arm. It cannot determine if the baby has a chromosomal disorder but can indicate whether you have a low or high risk of your baby having spina bifida or Down's syndrome. The test will detect about four out of five spina bifida pregnancies and about two out of three Down's syndrome pregnancies.

Diagnostic tests

Ultrasound scanning is used with chorionic villus sampling (**CVS**) and **amniocentesis**, so that the doctor can see the exact position of the baby and the placenta. Scans are also sometimes used to detect some abnormalities. (*See page 32 for more information about ultrasound scanning*).

The **CVS** check for chromosomal abnormalities, mainly Down's syndrome, and amniocentesis are tests which are usually only offered to women who have a higher risk of having a baby with a disability. An older mother, for example, is more likely to have a baby with Down's syndrome. A test may also be offered to a mother who has had a previous pregnancy affected by one of these abnormalities. There is a very small (about 2%) risk of miscarriage with these tests.

CVS can be performed from 11 weeks of pregnancy. A fine tube goes into the uterus, usually through the abdomen, and a syringe is used to remove a sample of the chorionic villus, the tissue forming the placenta. There is a 1–2% risk of miscarriage with this test. Results may be available after 48 hours but the results of a more detailed examination can take up to 14 days. The main advantage of CVS over aminocentesis is that CVS can be done earlier. A CVS may not be offered locally so you may be referred to a centre outside your area.

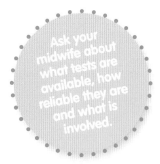

Ask your midwife about what tests are available, how reliable they are and what is involved.

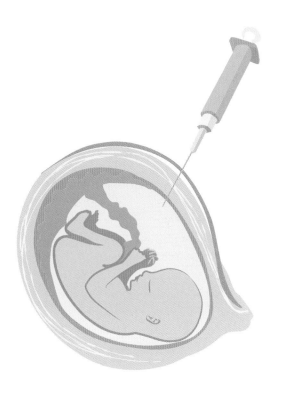

Amniocentesis is carried out after 15 weeks. A needle is inserted into the uterus through the abdomen and a sample of amniotic fluid is taken with a syringe.

There is a 1% risk of miscarriage, which will be discussed with you. Results will be available within 48 hours but the outcome of a detailed examination can take up to 21 days.

Down's syndrome and spina bifida

Down's syndrome: this describes people with an extra chromosome. Children with Down's syndrome will have learning difficulties and need help with their education. Although many have a healthy life, some have problems such as heart defects. Older mothers are more likely to have a baby with Down's syndrome. The risk rises from one in every 1,500 births for women aged 20 years, to one in every 900 births for women aged 30 years. It increases to one in every 100 births for women aged 40 years.

> You will receive further information on screening tests offered during pregnancy from your midwife and they will be happy to answer any questions.

Spina bifida: spina bifida and anencephaly are the two main types of condition known as neural tube defects, which affect about one in every 500 pregnancies.

Babies with spina bifida have an opening in the bones of the spine and the nerves to the lower part of the body are damaged. This can lead to problems with walking and with bowel and bladder control. Sometimes there can also be learning difficulties. The level of disability varies and many people with spina bifida lead fulfilling lives.

In babies with anencephaly, the skull and brain are not properly formed. These babies generally die before or soon after they are born.

Research has shown that taking 400 mcg of folic acid before conception and into the 12th week of pregnancy can reduce the risk of neural tube defects *(see page 6 for information on folic acid).*

Is there a problem?

When tests show there could be a problem, you need more information and support.

It's important to know what the test result shows, whether it's definite or not, and whether you need to make decisions about labour or birth or the future of your pregnancy.

> There can be disadvantages with antenatal tests. My blood test came back with a query, and further investigation was needed to rule out spina bifida. I was told there was probably nothing to worry about, but of course I did. Even though I was given the 'all clear', I think it increased my anxiety for nothing.
>
> *Fiona, Renfrewshire*

You may need time to consider your options. Support groups can help you with these difficult decisions *(see **Further help**, page 206)* and you can ask to talk with your midwife as well as your GP. If the tests indicate a disability, you may want to talk to parents who have a child with a similar condition to find out more about it. No one should try to influence you in any way; the decisions you make based on this information have to be yours and your partner's.

week 15-16

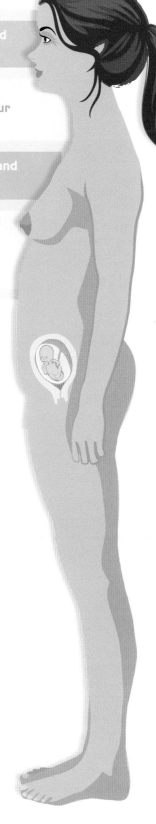

Your baby is becoming sensitive to light.

She's sucking her thumb in there, and all her joints and limbs can move.

You may have that pregnancy 'glow' – your hair looks thicker and your skin more plumped out.

Your 'bump' is probably starting to show, and your waist is disappearing!

Your ordinary clothes are feeling a bit tight.

Hopefully you're feeling less sick and your breasts may be less tender.

Your baby's body is growing faster to catch up with the size of her head.

Fine, downy hair called lanugo has started to grow on your baby's body, but this will disappear before birth.

It's just possible you've begun to feel the fetus inside you (quickening), although this may not happen for weeks yet.

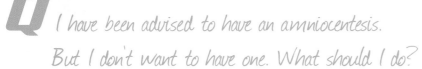

Q I have been advised to have an amniocentesis. But I don't want to have one. What should I do?

A. Only you can decide this. There is a small risk of miscarriage with amniocentesis and you may want to compare that with the risk of having a baby with an abnormality. Discuss the risks with your midwife. You may not want to terminate your pregnancy under any circumstances and, if so, there is no real reason to have an amniocentesis – though some parents want to know if their child will have a disability so they can prepare themselves for it. It is your right to decide whether to accept the offer of a test.

Twins and multiple births

The birth of more than one baby is always known as a multiple birth, whether there are two, three or more. One baby at a time is known as a singleton.

Multiple birth – the statistics:

○ one pregnancy in every 80 is a twin pregnancy

○ one pregnancy in 8,000 is triplets

○ one pregnancy in 800,000 is quads.

Twins – how pregnancy and birth are different

Twins (and more) are formed either by the egg splitting shortly after fertilisation (identical twins) or by two or more eggs being fertilised by two or more sperm (non-identical or fraternal twins). Non-identical twins are slightly more likely to happen after a course of fertility treatment which stimulates ovulation, and which means more than one egg may be released. They can also happen when more than one fertilised egg is put into the uterus after in vitro fertilisation (IVF – test-tube pregnancy).

Twins will show up on the screen during an ultrasound scan. They may be suspected if your uterus is larger than expected at this stage of pregnancy.

The main concern with a multiple pregnancy, even if you are healthy and have no major problems, is that the minor discomforts of pregnancy may be heightened. That means (for example) more backache, fatigue, heartburn and nausea, constipation and piles. The increased weight gain and the excess of pregnancy hormones contribute to this. You'll need lots of rest, especially later on in pregnancy and a healthy diet is particularly important *(see pages 14–17).*

Extra care

If you are expecting twins, or more, you will receive more attention during pregnancy.

The reasons for extra care include:

• a greater risk of high blood pressure, which needs careful observation and possible treatment

• the fact that twins, or more, are likely to be born before 40 weeks – 37 or 38 weeks is average for twins, but 25% of twin pregnancies lead to birth before 36 weeks

• a greater likelihood of birth problems

• Caesarean section which may be necessary to speed up delivery or to deliver the second twin quickly – less space in the uterus means one or both twins may be in a difficult, or impossible, position for a vaginal birth.

Triplet pregnancy is even more likely than twin pregnancy to end in a preterm or operative delivery (or both). Caesarean section is considered virtually inevitable for quads or quintuplets to control the delivery. Even so, while multiple pregnancy is hard work, and a multiple labour and delivery may be more of a challenge to everyone, especially you, the majority of twin and triplet births are as joyous and rewarding as any other, and many pregnancies and births are perfectly straightforward.

For some women, being told that they are expecting twins or triplets may come as a real shock and they may find it hard to cope

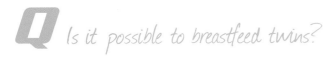

Q Is it possible to breastfeed twins?

A. Yes it certainly is! Your body will make as much milk as your babies need. Mothers can even breastfeed triplets.

You will receive help to learn how to hold your babies so they can attach well and feed effectively. If they are small you may need extra help while they gradually get better at feeding.

Twins tend to differ in their feeding habits, just as any other two babies may, and keeping them both happy may be hard in the early weeks. You need to feel confident, and to have encouragement from the people around you. You'll also need help with other jobs in the house. In time, feeding becomes less intensive – and many women find breastfeeding easier than making up bottles of formula milk.

with the thought of looking after more than one baby. You will need all the support you can get. There is special support for twin and multiple birth families and you should ask your midwife about local groups *(see **Further help**, page 205)*. You will need plenty of help once your babies are born with things like bathing and nappy changing.

Twins in the uterus – how do they lie?

The best presentation of twins is with both lying head-down – 'cephalic' or 'vertex' – and this is the most common. However, pressure on space in the uterus means it's also quite common for one or both babies to be breech (feet or bottom down). A transverse lie (baby across the uterus) is also a possibility and, if this is the case with the first presenting twin, a Caesarean section is inevitable. If the first twin has been born vaginally but the second twin is lying across the uterus, there may be an attempt to turn the second twin.

at a glance

✵ If you're pregnant with twins (or more!) you'll get extra care.

✵ The main concern is that you may have increased discomfort such as backache, or go into labour early.

✵ A healthy diet is particularly important – as is lots of rest.

See TAMBA – the Twins and Multiple Birth Association for more information, www.tamba.org.uk and visit www.laleche.org.uk for tips on breastfeeding.

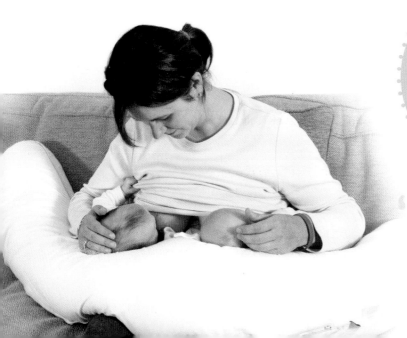

I was worried about how I would manage to breastfeed twins, but breastfeeding my girls has been a fantastic experience and because there is so much help and support out there it's actually easier than making up feeds!
Miriam, Edinburgh

Antenatal classes

You have the opportunity to attend antenatal classes before the birth. These are also called 'childbirth education' or 'preparation for parenthood' classes.

Good antenatal classes help you prepare for labour, birth and early parenthood with confidence.

Why go to an antenatal class?

Most clinics, hospitals and health centres have antenatal classes. They are free and usually run by midwives, with possible input from other health professionals. Antenatal classes are a good way to meet people who, like you, are about to become parents. Some lifelong friendships have been formed while practising breathing techniques! Classes also cover looking after yourself and your baby after birth.

Other non-NHS classes may charge a fee and are usually run by specially trained antenatal teachers, often in their own home.

There's more information in **Further help**.

Antenatal classes aim to prepare you and your partner (or whoever will be supporting you at the birth) for what's to come.

They cover all sorts of things that you may have questions about, such as:

- health in pregnancy including advice on diet and how to cope with minor discomforts

- what to expect in later pregnancy – including the early signs of labour

- what to expect during labour and birth and pain relief options

- techniques such as relaxation and breathing to help you cope with labour and birth

- possible problems during labour, and interventions such as Caesarean section

- exercises for before, during and after labour

- birth plans

- feeding and caring for your baby safely.

Some classes are specially designed for different groups of women, such as teenage mums or mums from the same ethnic groups. Your midwife can tell you what's going on in your area.

week 17-18

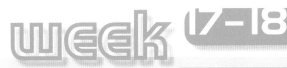

She is about 13 cm (a little more than 5 inches) from the top of her head to her bottom.

Your baby's kidneys have started producing urine, most of which travels through the placenta for your body to deal with.

You may be able to hear your baby's heart beating when you're examined.

You may feel her move round – but it's nothing to worry about if you don't feel anything yet.

Her tastebuds are beginning to form.

Your baby can kick and move around and is probably doing it a lot, particularly at night when your movement isn't rocking her to sleep.

When to go?

Antenatal classes usually run in two to six sessions towards the end of your pregnancy. It may be a good idea to book earlier, however, so that you get a place in a class that suits you. Some areas run 'early classes' where things like looking after yourself in pregnancy, exercise and common problems are discussed.

Who should I go with?

It's up to you. Discuss this with your partner to find out how they feel about going. Some classes are run for women only and some for couples.

There's nothing to stop you taking a friend along for support if you feel uncomfortable going alone. Female friends and relatives often accompany women to classes.

Bringing your partner gives them a chance to ask questions, to meet others who may share their concerns and to learn how to support you at the birth and during breastfeeding. You can practise relaxation and breathing techniques with them too.

at a glance

* Your midwife can tell you what's available locally.

* Antenatal classes do more than give information – they're also a good way to meet people.

* It's up to you and your partner whether you both go along.

* Most antenatal classes encourage dads and partners and there may be a special session just for them.

Safety during lambing season

Coming into close contact with sheep during lambing may risk your own health, and the health of your unborn child, from infections that can occur in some ewes. While pregnant you should avoid close contact with sheep during the lambing season.

While the number of reported infections and human miscarriages resulting from contact with sheep is extremely small, pregnant women need to be aware of the potential risks. If you do become ill (experience fever or flu-like symptoms) and are concerned that you could have acquired infection from a farm environment, you should seek immediate medical advice.

What to **wear** when you're pregnant

After about four or five months you'll find that you don't fit into your normal clothes because your waist has thickened and your breasts are larger. But you don't need to splash out on lots of expensive new clothes that you may never wear again.

What to look for

Lots of department stores and boutiques carry maternity lines now and they don't all cost the earth. Just buy the size you normally take when you're not pregnant.

Most women find it more comfortable to wear a bra, even if they don't normally wear one. Many midwives and retail outlets advise against wearing underwired bras during pregnancy as the rigid wiring structure may interfere with the natural changes in the size and shape of your breasts. This may in turn 'squash' developing milk ducts. You may need to be measured two or three times during pregnancy – just be aware of whether or not the bra you are wearing is comfortable and supportive. Nursing bras have cups which unhook or unzip and are helpful for breastfeeding later.

Even if you normally love high heels, you may find you're more comfortable in flatter 'sensible' shoes while you're pregnant. Fluid retention can make your ankles swell and feel uncomfortable, and your centre of gravity is changing, so heels can put a strain on your lower back.

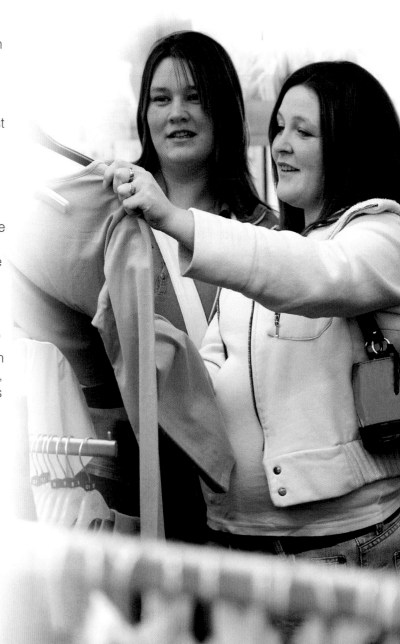

> **I got a lot of maternity clothes from my sister and best friend and didn't need to buy anything until my last month.**
> *Kirsty, Elgin*

week 19

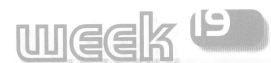

You're about halfway there; you may feel excited or scared or both.

Your baby's beginning to form her second teeth, behind the first ones.

You could be feeling hungrier – carry healthy snacks like fruit to deal with those pangs.

At about this time your baby's body starts being covered with 'vernix', a greasy substance which coats her skin, forming a waterproof layer.

Your back may be sore, you may feel more tired and you could feel slightly breathless.

Sex during pregnancy

Sex is normally perfectly safe in pregnancy. Any sexual activity that doesn't harm you will not harm your baby. You don't risk hurting or affecting your baby.

Is it ever risky?

Your baby is protected in the uterus by the bag of waters, which cushions movement. Your baby may feel the movements of vigorous sexual activity, but they won't do her any harm. Occasionally, women who have had a number of miscarriages may be advised not to have sex around the time their period would have been due, or even not at all during the first three months. There's no evidence that sex and miscarriage are linked though, and some doctors disagree about how to advise couples in this situation.

○ Some women feel that sex with either the man or woman on top is a little uncomfortable in later pregnancy. You can get round this by the person on top bearing their weight on their arms. Or try side-by-side positions.

○ Some women – and some men – get less keen on penetrative sex as the pregnancy develops. That's fine. You can have closeness and as much sexual excitement as you want without it.

Women and men sometimes find their desire for sex changes during pregnancy, and both may go off it. This is not serious or long-lasting. Keep your closeness with lots of warm, physical contact that need not lead to sex. If sex played an important role in your lives before, then the feelings are very likely to come back in time.

at a glance

✻ Most women can have sex while they are pregnant.

✻ You may even find you enjoy it more than usual at some stages of pregnancy.

✻ It's important to talk about it with your partner.

> I didn't like to ask my partner if she wanted to make love because I thought it might harm the baby. So I was really glad when she suggested it.
>
> *Andrew, Galashiels*

Minor problems in pregnancy

At around week 20 you might start to show that so-called pregnancy 'glow'. However, even if you are experiencing a healthy and trouble-free pregnancy there are minor troubles that can affect you – though these are often mild and short-lived.

How to cope

Don't keep your worries to yourself. Your midwife or GP will advise and reassure you about how to deal with most of the less serious discomforts of pregnancy.

Backache can get worse as you get further along. There is extra strain on your joints and hips as you put on more weight and get closer to the birth. Gentle exercise and taking care while lifting can make a big difference as well as:

- wearing flats or shoes with a low heel
- sitting and standing with your back straight and your shoulders relaxed
- bending at the knees and avoiding lifting heavy weights.

Bleeding gums happen when gums become swollen because of plaque deposits. During pregnancy, due to hormonal effects, even a small build-up of plaque can cause irritation to the gums. This is called 'pregnancy gingivitis'. Brushing twice daily with fluoride toothpaste and regular flossing can help prevent gingivitis. Visit your dentist regularly.

Constipation can be a problem in pregnancy due to all the changes taking place in your body and new hormones rushing around. Your diet can be the best way to tackle constipation; eat plenty of fibre-rich food – vegetables, fruit, beans and wholegrain bread – and make sure you are getting enough fluids. Moderate exercise, like swimming or walking, can also help you stay regular.

Cystitis is a urine infection which may cause a burning sensation when you pee and make you feel you need to pass urine all the time – but these symptoms can often be felt in pregnancy anyway. If you have symptoms like this, discuss them with your midwife. You may be given a course of safe antibiotics if there is an infection.

Heartburn (indigestion) is a burning sensation around the breastbone. It is more common in later pregnancy. Strong tea or coffee, pure fruit juice, spicy and fatty foods can make it feel worse. Take your time when you eat.

Piles or haemorrhoids are varicose veins of the back passage, or anus. They are sometimes very painful and itchy, and they can be made worse by constipation. Your midwife or GP can advise on treatment.

Swelling of the ankles, fingers, face and hands is also called oedema and happens because the body holds more fluid in pregnancy (a certain amount is normal in later pregnancy). More severe cases can indicate pre-eclampsia, if present with other signs *(see page 79)*.

Sometimes fluid collects in the wrists, producing a painful or tingling sensation in the fingers. This is called 'carpal tunnel syndrome'. If it is very troublesome, speak to your midwife or GP.

week 20

Congratulations, you are halfway though your pregnancy!

Your baby is about 16.5 cm (6½ inches) from her head to her bottom. She's 25.5 cm (10 inches) from head to toe.

She is very active – before she gets too big to whirl around in the uterus.

You may be able to feel your baby move now – although probably nobody else can.

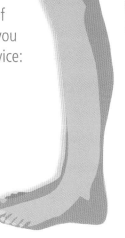

Varicose veins are swollen veins, usually in the legs, but sometimes in the vulva (vaginal opening) too. They may cause aching and sometimes itching. Support tights can help. Avoid standing for long periods and try to rest with your legs up when you can. Always tell your midwife or GP if you notice any hot, red or painful areas in your legs or vulva.

Certain exercises can help – ask your midwife, an obstetric physiotherapist or your antenatal teacher.

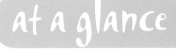

at a glance

✳ Most problems you'll have in pregnancy aren't serious for you or your baby.

✳ Don't suffer in silence – talk to your midwife or GP.

✳ Remember all NHS dental treatment is free during pregnancy and for one year after the birth.

Unasked-for advice can be one of the worst irritants of pregnancy! Now that you are really starting to show you may find these tips helpful for handling unwanted advice:

- take it with a grain of salt – advice is usually well-meant and shows that they care

- trust yourself and your instincts – you know how you feel better than anyone

- say thank you and carry on!

Rely on trusted sources of information like your midwife or GP, and ask them if you have questions.

More serious complications in pregnancy

If you are at all concerned contact your midwife, GP or NHS 24.

Changes in your body because of pregnancy can lead to minor health problems such as backache or varicose veins. You may need treatment, or careful observation, if there are signs of more serious problems in your pregnancy. These problems include:

Anaemia

Anaemia is a condition which occurs when there are not enough red blood cells in your body. The condition shows up in a blood test. Anaemia may be the result of illness, poor diet, severe sickness or extra strain on your body, such as when you are expecting twins. You will be given information on changing your diet, and you may be prescribed iron and vitamin supplements.

Vaginal bleeding

You should get medical advice straight away if you are bleeding from the vagina in pregnancy, or if you experience severe abdominal pain. Sometimes the placenta is lying so low it covers the cervix. It is more likely to bleed in this position. This condition – placenta praevia – is uncommon and needs careful observation. In later pregnancy, it could be that the placenta is separating from the uterine wall. This could be life threatening to you and your baby. Not all instances of bleeding are serious – some women do bleed a little, on and off, throughout pregnancy, for a variety of minor reasons. Discuss any bleeding with your midwife.

Continued sickness

There are various reasons for this, including a twin pregnancy or being particularly sensitive to hormones. If you are unfortunate, the pregnancy sickness that usually disappears at around 12 weeks persists into later pregnancy. Very severe cases, known as hyperemesis gravidarum, need hospital treatment.

Diabetes

Some women develop diabetes during pregnancy. The condition disappears after pregnancy, although some women do go on to develop diabetes later. The pregnancy may be affected, as the baby tends to get larger, and the diabetes will be monitored to make sure it remains under control. You may need to attend a different antenatal clinic and see a specialist obstetrician.

High blood pressure

Your blood pressure is checked regularly at the antenatal clinic. When blood pressure is very high, it can be diagnosed as pregnancy-induced hypertension. If it's present with other symptoms, it can be a sign of pre-eclampsia (see page 79). High blood pressure can affect your health and that of your growing baby.

Itching

Occasionally women develop a severe itching of the skin in pregnancy. This is usually no more than an irritating discomfort – but occasionally it can be the sign of a condition called obstetric cholestasis, where the liver is affected by pregnancy. See your midwife if your itch doesn't clear up, or if no treatment helps.

Pelvic girdle pain

This happens when the small joint (the symphysis pubis) at the front of the bony girdle of the pelvis opens up too far. It can cause a lot of pain when walking or even standing. Physiotherapy or wearing a support belt can help (see **Further help**, page 206).

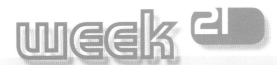

week 21

Your baby's eyebrows and eyelashes are growing.

Due to disturbed sleep you may get a bit absent-minded and forget things.

You may start getting indigestion.

You may have a second routine ultrasound (depending on what part of the country you live in). Some areas only offer a second scan if there appears to be a problem.

Your baby can hear sounds both inside and outside your body – if you chat to her she will get to know your voice.

Q *My baby isn't growing very well. Is this serious?*

A. It may be, but some babies are naturally small, and some catch up in later pregnancy. Your dates may be incorrect, so you may not be as far on in your pregnancy as you think. It's very difficult to diagnose accurately if a baby isn't growing well. Most small babies are born healthy and grow into normal healthy children.

Some babies have intrauterine growth retardation (IUGR), which means they are smaller and lighter than most babies at that stage of pregnancy. IUGR may happen because the placenta isn't nourishing the baby well, or perhaps because the baby has an underlying condition which is preventing growth. If the mother's diet is very poor or she is a smoker this can cause poor growth in the baby. Occasionally, poor growth in the baby can be a sign of pre-eclampsia in the mother.

at a glance

✳ Most babies are born healthy.

✳ There are tests that can help measure your baby's development more accurately.

✳ Sometimes you can develop problems which can affect you or your unborn baby.

✳ You may have to go into hospital, but many conditions are treated at home by community midwives or GPs.

Emotions: how you and your partner may be feeling

There's no 'normal' way to feel while you're pregnant, and everyone is different.

Pregnancy is an emotional time

You may not have planned the pregnancy and, especially if you're on your own, may wonder how you'll cope. Even if you were desperate to have a baby, now you're actually expecting one you can feel worried, apprehensive and downright scared.

Then again, you may find that you're overjoyed a lot of the time and can't help smiling, even when you're suffering with morning sickness!

Even if you're not the sort of person who cries a lot, that can change in pregnancy. Possibly the slightest thing will set you off, ranging from a sad report on the news to, believe it or not, the most ordinary scene in your favourite soap.

Other women find they get really irritable, tense and moody – which can be difficult for those closest to them.

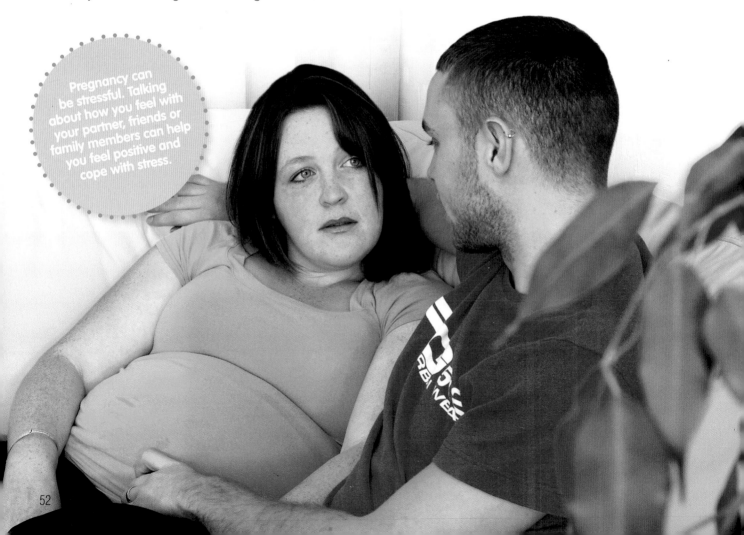

Pregnancy can be stressful. Talking about how you feel with your partner, friends or family members can help you feel positive and cope with stress.

week 22
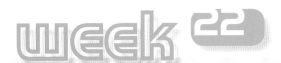

Your baby has probably reached the grand weight of one pound (about 500 g).

Your baby will probably be pretty active down there and may kick in response to certain sounds, such as your voice.

This may be the time when it really sinks in that you and your partner are going to be parents.

She can grasp with her hands and may grip the umbilical cord.

Depression and pregnancy

Around 1 in 10 women will have mild to moderate depression during pregnancy. Those who have suffered it before can be at particular risk.

However you're feeling, there's no need to suffer in silence. Talk to your midwife who will be able to suggest ways you can feel better.

It's a good idea to share your feelings with your partner too. He or she may be feeling lots of the same things. It's a huge thing having a baby and it will change your lives. While that is really exciting it's natural to feel nervous too. You may wonder what sort of parents you'll be. You may also find that, if you had problems in your own childhood, thoughts of this come flooding back, even though you've pushed them to the back of your mind for years.

You are not alone

You may also worry about losing your sense of who you are – of being you. While you're getting loads of attention at this time in your life – lots of appointments, people being excited for you – you may feel that it's the baby who's the focus of attention, not you. Your partner may feel shut out if he or she thinks all you're thinking about is the baby.

You'll both know that your life will be different after the baby is born. You'll be responsible for someone else, and you'll have to look after their needs. Going to the cinema or the pub will take planning – you won't be able to do things on the spur of the moment anymore.

All these worries are normal and it may help to talk to others who've been through it. Your midwife may be able to suggest parenting groups or you may meet people in a similar situation at antenatal classes *(see page 44–45).*

at a glance

✳ Expecting a baby can make you and your partner feel over the moon with joy or terrified – or both at the same time.

✳ Your body is surging with all sorts of hormones which affect your feelings.

✳ Even without the 'pregnancy hormones' your partner is going through many of the same uncertainties and feelings as you.

✳ You're doing an amazing thing and it's not surprising that you feel a bit overwhelmed.

It's natural to have worries about things such as whether your baby will be OK, how you'll cope with the birth, breastfeeding, going back to work and money matters.

Weight gain and other changes to your body

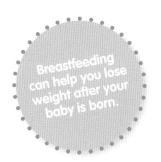

Breastfeeding can help you lose weight after your baby is born.

If you've always watched your weight, it can feel strange to get on the scales and see that your weight keeps going up. Even though, logically, you know it has to, you can still feel a bit funny about it. The fact is that slow, gradual weight gain is the sign of a healthy pregnancy.

How the weight is made up

- baby: 2.5–4 kg (5–9 lbs)
- placenta: 0.5–1 kg (1–2 lbs)
- amniotic fluid: 1.5–2.5 kg (3–5 lbs)
- increased blood volume and fluids (yours): 2–4 kg (4–9 lbs)
- extra weight of uterus, breasts and fat and protein stores: 2–5 kg (4–11 lbs).

You'll be weighed at the beginning of your pregnancy so that the midwives or obstetricians have something to compare your weight to as the pregnancy develops.

Most weight gain is in the middle part of the pregnancy (four to seven months), although you may find you put on a fair bit near the start because of fluid retention. Some women don't gain any weight at all in the last two to three weeks.

Your midwife will be keeping an eye out for rapid weight gain in the last ten weeks of pregnancy as this can be one of the signs of pre-eclampsia, which is serious (see page 79).

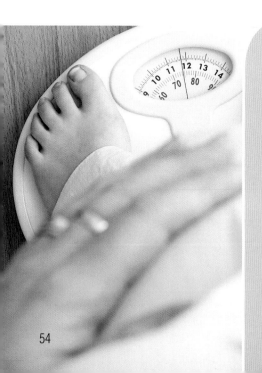

Healthy weight gain

There is not a 'right' amount of weight to put on as it will vary from woman to woman, depending on things like height, body shape and the weight you were when you got pregnant. Experts say that you can expect to put on between 9 and 16 kg (19 and 35 lbs) during your pregnancy (provided you're not expecting more than one baby). The average is about 12.5 kg (28 lbs).

Only about a third of the extra weight is due to the baby, amniotic fluid and placenta. The rest is the extra weight you need to support the pregnancy and prepare for what happens afterwards.

Healthy eating

As you move through your pregnancy, you may find you get hungrier, especially between meals, so it can be tempting to reach for the crisps and chocolate. Now and again this is OK, but you may find it useful to carry healthy snacks around with you to satisfy your food cravings and avoid temptation *(see page 16)*.

It's important to eat well during pregnancy to give your baby the best start in life *(see page 14)*.

You should aim to have about eight glasses of water a day, jazz it up with ice and a slice of lemon. Or try diluted fruit juice or very weak cordial.

Pelvic floor exercises

Around now you may begin to realise why you should be doing pelvic floor exercises (in other words, you may have a little leak of urine!). Doing them now is important to get those vital muscles in trim for the rest of your pregnancy and beyond. *(See **Pelvic floor exercises**, page 147)*.

Stretch marks

You may develop stretch marks, thin lines on the skin caused by collagen (the thing that makes our skin elastic and stretchy) tearing as your body expands to cope with pregnancy. These can look quite red but will fade to become faint, silvery lines afterwards. A healthy diet and not putting on weight too quickly may help.

at a glance

❋ The 'right' amount of weight for you may not be the same as for someone else.

❋ Keeping fit and healthy in pregnancy is good for you and your baby.

other physical changes

- Your skin may show some changes. You may find you develop skin tags, which are little bits of extra skin, particularly at points where your clothing is rubbing. These are nothing to worry about.

- You may suffer from rashes or spots. Wearing cotton clothing may ease heat rashes.

- You may find your nipples, freckles and moles get darker.

Planning ahead

There is a lot to think about in the coming months and having the right information can help you make some important decisions. Your midwife will be happy to answer questions as your pregnancy progresses.

Talking about breastfeeding

During pregnancy your midwife will discuss the health benefits of breastfeeding for both you and your baby, to make sure you have all the information you need to make your choice. Some areas run breastfeeding workshops which you can attend when you are pregnant. They give you lots of information about what breastfeeding is like and what you can expect in the early days.

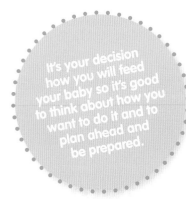

It's your decision how you will feed your baby so it's good to think about how you want to do it and to plan ahead and be prepared.

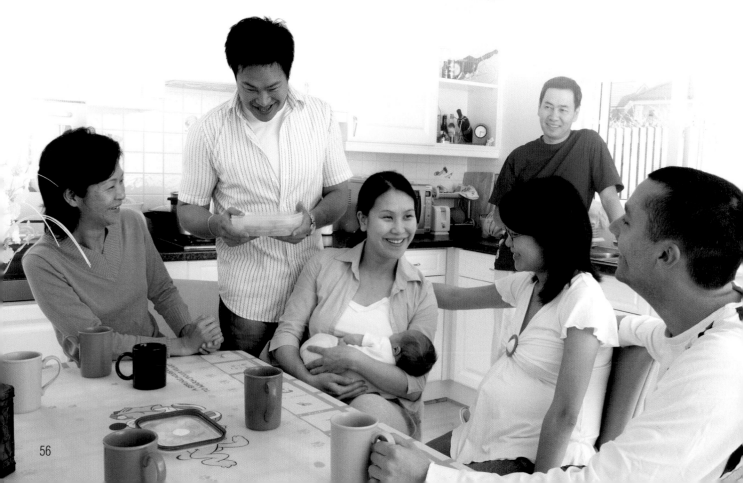

Reasons to breastfeed

Breastfeeding protects your baby's health from birth. Research also shows that the benefits can last into childhood and beyond. Breast milk builds immunity to infection, and can help prevent obesity and childhood-onset diabetes.

Health benefits

You will be told about the health benefits of breastfeeding for you and your baby. This is not to press you to breastfeed, but to make sure you have all the information you need to make your choice. It can be helpful to talk to other breastfeeding mums and find out what kind of support is there for you.

Breastfed babies are less likely to have many illnesses, including:

○ Chest, urine, ear and gastro-intestinal infections (sickness and diarrhoea). They have better immunity and protection because of the antibodies and anti-infective properties in breast milk. Formula milk cannot copy these.

○ Wheezing when breathing, asthma, eczema, allergies and diabetes, particularly where this runs in the family. Formula milk is made from cow's milk which may cause some sensitive babies to develop these conditions.

○ High blood pressure and obesity. Many breastfed babies have better appetite control.

Breastfed babies often have improved eyesight and increased alertness because special fats found in breast milk are good for their rapidly growing brains.

In addition, breast milk has special value for sick and premature babies, protecting them against infections and serious gut problems.

Breastfeeding has benefits for you too

Mothers who breastfeed have a lower risk of:

- ovarian and breast cancer

- hip fracture in later life, caused by the bone disease osteoporosis.

Breastfeeding may also help you return to your pre-pregnancy weight. In pregnancy, your body lays down fat stores for breastfeeding. If you breastfeed, you use these stores, helping to avoid the long-term health risks associated with being overweight, such as diabetes, high blood pressure, cancer and heart disease.

Although it's a natural process, you and your baby will both need to learn how to breastfeed. For some mothers it may be difficult for the first few weeks. It helps to be prepared for it and have the support of people around you, including your midwife and your family.

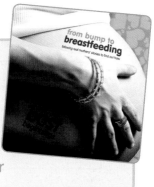

This free DVD from NHS Health Scotland will give you the information you need to begin and continue breastfeeding. Ask your midwife for a copy.

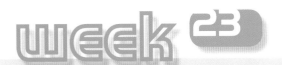
week 23

You may be suffering backache, varicose veins or leg cramps (see pages 48–49).

Your baby has skin but no fat so she looks a bit wrinkly.

Her hearing is well established and she can make out certain noises such as a rumbling stomach, your heartbeat and noises such as the vacuum cleaner.

Your baby will gain weight rapidly over the next four weeks.

How your choice to breastfeed is supported

As soon as your baby is born you will start the bonding process (getting to know and love your baby) by enjoying skin-to-skin contact with her. This keeps your baby warm and calms her by stabilising her heartbeat and breathing. It also helps to stimulate your breastfeeding hormones.

Rooming in

Most maternity units in hospitals now recommend that babies stay with their mums 24 hours a day. This is called 'rooming in' and it helps you to get used to breastfeeding your baby as well as reducing the risk of infection. You'll have support on hand from the staff in the maternity ward – as well as other new mums – and, of course, you'll have the opportunity to spend time with your new baby and start bonding with her.

Help and advice

When you are in hospital – and once you are back at home – your midwife will be on hand to give you plenty of practical advice to help you to establish breastfeeding. You'll be shown how to hold your baby (positioning) and how to encourage her to take your nipple and breast in her mouth correctly (attachment). This will help your baby to feed effectively – and also help you to avoid sore nipples or some of the other problems that new mums can experience when breastfeeding for the first time.

Early first feeds

When you start breastfeeding your baby, the first milk she gets will be colostrum. This will help her to have her first bowel movements and, as it is rich in antibodies, will also help her to fight infections.

Exclusive breastfeeding

Experts now believe that it is best to avoid bottles and teats altogether if you want to breastfeed successfully. Your midwife will be happy to discuss this with you.

Baby-led feeding

By allowing your baby to feed according to her own hunger or thirst – rather than a rigid timetable – you'll find that you establish a good supply of milk and avoid breast engorgement.

For further information and advice on breastfeeding, refer to pages 122–125 in this book – or talk to your midwife to discuss your choice to breastfeed.

Ask your midwife for your free copy of NHS Health Scotland's *Off to a good start* for more information on breastfeeding your baby.

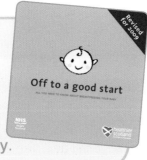

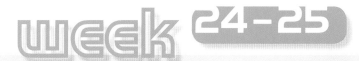

week 24-25

You may be feeling less tired and more energetic.

Your baby's lungs aren't completely mature yet but she is practising making breathing movements.

If you are constipated, eating fibre-rich food such as wholemeal bread, having lots of fruit and drinking plenty of water can help, so can a bit of exercise – try taking a brisk walk.

Your baby is viable – that is, some babies born at this stage have gone on to survive.

Vitamin K and your new baby

Vitamin K occurs naturally in food, especially in some vegetables. We all need vitamin K to help make our blood clot, preventing bleeding. When babies are born they have very little vitamin K, and very rarely, a small number of babies may start to bleed because of this.

Vitamin K supplements

Vitamin K supplements are offered straight after birth so it's important to think about it beforehand. Your midwife or hospital doctor will be able to give you information about it but it's up to you whether to go ahead with it. Health experts recommend that all new babies receive vitamin K shortly after they are born to remove the small risk that they will start bleeding.

There are two methods of giving vitamin K: by injection, which is done in one dose; or by mouth, which means the baby will need several doses. If it's given by mouth, it is recommended that all babies get two doses within the first week. For babies who are exclusively breastfed, a third dose will be given at one month. Babies who have formula milk won't need the third dose, because formula milk already contains vitamin K. It is important that all the doses are given to make sure the baby is protected. Remember, however, that breastfeeding your baby is the best choice for all-round health.

Bleeding or bruising at any time in the first six months must be looked at urgently as it can be a sign of vitamin K deficiency bleeding. Babies need to be seen by their GP or health visitor/public health nurse if their stools are pale and their urine is dark.

at a glance

✳ Breastfeeding gets your baby off to the best possible start – it is good for both of you!

✳ There is lots of support for you, both before and after your baby is born.

✳ Ask your midwife if you have any questions about the benefits of breastfeeding.

✳ Attending a breastfeeding workshop while you are still pregnant can give you a good idea of what to expect.

✳ You'll have to make a decision about vitamin K immediately after birth so think about it now.

✳ Your midwife will provide information about vitamin K and will be happy to answer any questions.

Travel during pregnancy

All the usual precautions of travelling apply as a pregnant traveller but avoiding hassles and stress can be even more acute. Whether you are travelling for holiday, work or for family events try and minimise potential difficulties by bringing a copy of your antenatal notes and if you are leaving the country make sure you are covered by medical insurance.

Holidays and travel by plane

If you're planning a holiday while you're pregnant, the best time is the middle trimester (weeks 13–26). By this time, the queasiness of early pregnancy should be passing and the risk of miscarriage has fallen.

Remember to take your maternity notes with you whenever you're away from home for a couple of days or longer, in case you need to seek medical help.

Most airlines won't let you fly if you are within about a month of your due date, and some will require a letter from your GP saying you're fit to fly when you're seven months pregnant. Check with the airline before you book.

Check with your midwife or GP that there's no medical reason to stop you flying, such as high blood pressure or a predisposition to deep vein thrombosis *(see box opposite)* and that you can safely get all the vaccinations you need. Some vaccinations are not recommended during pregnancy, particularly in the first three months.

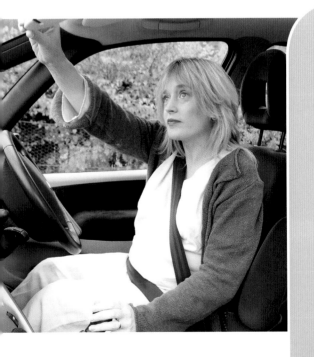

In the car

There's nothing to stop you driving or being a passenger in a car while you're pregnant. For safety reasons, it's important that you wear a seatbelt as normal. The lap strap should go across the hips, fitting comfortably under the bump, while the diagonal strap should be placed between the breasts around the bump. Don't put either strap across the bump.

In the last few weeks of your pregnancy you may not want to drive — your bump may get in the way!

coping with jet lag

The normal problems of jet lag; disrupted sleep, dehydration, stiffness and minor aches and pains, can be even worse for pregnant women. Bear this in mind when planning a trip during your pregnancy and try to avoid long-haul flights. If you are travelling by plane remember to:

- give yourself plenty of time to adjust to local times

- recognise it may take you a bit longer than before to adjust once you are home again

- take healthy snacks with you for the flight so you can follow your own eating schedule

- bring whatever comfort aids you are used to: an extra pillow, head rest or warm socks can make a big difference

- drink plenty of water! You are much more susceptible to dehydration while flying so be sure to keep your fluid levels up.

Other things to consider

○ Healthcare cover in Europe is now covered by the European Health Insurance Card (EHIC). This replaced the old E111 form and is valid for three to five years. You can apply for this online at **www.dh.gov.uk/travellers**

○ Give some thought to where you go. The things you may normally love on holiday – like hot sunny weather – may not be a great idea if you're feeling uncomfortable and finding it difficult to sleep.

○ Non-essential travel to malaria areas is not recommended.

○ Special travel insurance which covers medical costs and allows you to cancel for pregnancy-related reasons is a must, as most insurance policies do not cover the consequences of pregnancy.

Deep vein thrombosis

There's been a lot of publicity linking long-haul flights with deep vein thrombosis, a condition in which a potentially dangerous blood clot forms. It's true that you're slightly more at risk when you're pregnant.

If you're worried about it, talk to your midwife who may recommend circulation-boosting stockings.

at a glance

❋ The best time to take a holiday or travel is in your second trimester – between your 13th and 26th week.

❋ Remember to take your maternity notes with you on holiday or whenever you are away for more than a couple of days.

❋ Make sure you have travel insurance which covers medical costs.

Lots of active holiday pursuits are probably fine – like walking and swimming. Talk to your midwife if you have questions.

Maternity leave and other benefits and payments

If you have a job, you've probably already been thinking about what you plan to do after your baby is born. You may want to return as soon as you can, you may want to go part-time or you may want to take a longer break from paid employment.

Maternity leave

All mothers who are employees are entitled to take Ordinary Maternity Leave (OML) and Additional Maternity Leave (AML). Statutory Maternity Pay (SMP) is currently 39 weeks from when the woman goes on OML. As a pregnant employee you are entitled to take up to one year's (52 weeks) maternity leave. This is made up of 26 weeks OML – during which your contract of employment continues – and 26 weeks AML – during which your contract of employment continues, but only certain terms of that contract apply. You and your employer may agree between yourselves for other terms to continue, but this is not required by law. There cannot be a gap between OML and AML.

You must tell your employer you intend to take maternity leave by the end of the 15th week before your expected week of delivery (EWD), unless this is not possible.

You can change your mind about when you want to start your leave providing you tell your employer at least 28 days in advance (unless this is not practical).

Your employer must respond to notification of your leave plans within 28 days unless you have varied that date, in which case your employer must respond within 28 days of the start of maternity leave.

Your job is protected. It's against the law for your employer to dismiss you or make you redundant for any reason connected with your pregnancy, the birth or maternity leave.

This is the case even if you are part-time, and it doesn't depend on how long you've worked for the employer.

Check your contract of employment or with your human resources department or trade union representative to find out what you're entitled to. Some employers offer better and more flexible maternity rights than those given by law.

Benefits payments

Working out the money that is due to you during and after pregnancy is quite complicated and things can change. For up-to-date advice check with your employer, your trade union or your local Citizens Advice Bureau. Visit the Citizens Advice Scotland website, **www.cas.org.uk** for more information. The most up-to-date information on benefits can also be found at **www.direct.gov.uk**

Statutory maternity pay (SMP)

Your employer must pay you SMP if you qualify (to see if you do, check the website referenced below). You'll receive 90% of your average earnings for the first six weeks and then a flat rate for the rest of the time (unless the 90% rate is less than the flat rate in which case you'll get this for the whole time). This flat rate varies so it's best to check it for yourself. Tax and National Insurance are payable on SMP. Visit **www.dwp.gov.uk** for up-to-date information.

To qualify for SMP you will need to have worked for your employer for 26 weeks by the 15th week before your baby is due and earn over the National Insurance lower earnings limit.

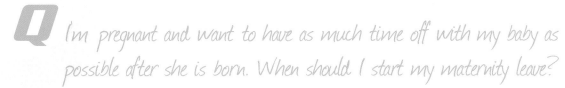

Q *I'm pregnant and want to have as much time off with my baby as possible after she is born. When should I start my maternity leave?*

A. You cannot start your maternity leave until 11 weeks before the baby is due. In theory you can work right up to the day the baby is born, and take all your leave after the birth.

In practice, you may feel you need to leave work a few weeks before the due date. Everyone feels differently and it is your decision.

Maternity allowance

If you do not qualify for SMP, for instance because your earnings are too low or you are self-employed, you can claim maternity allowance from the Benefits Agency. Maternity allowance will be paid at the flat rate of £100 per week (or 90% of average weekly earnings if this is less) for 26 weeks. To claim, you will need form MA1 from the Benefits Agency.

Parental leave

Both parents have the right to take up to 13 weeks unpaid parental leave per parent per child (18 weeks if the child is entitled to Disability Living Allowance). You must have worked for your employer for one year by the date you wish to take it. You can take parental leave after maternity or paternity leave, providing you give 21 days notice and the child is aged up to five years (or 18 days notice if the child is disabled).

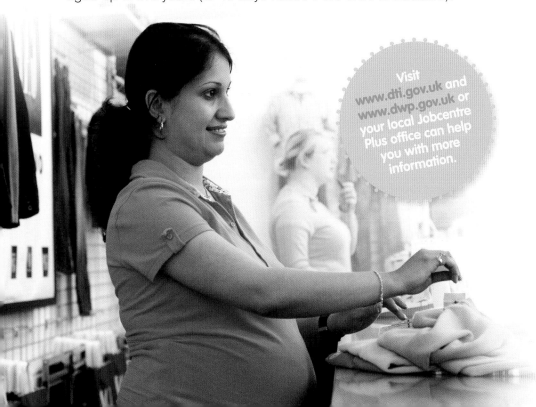

Visit www.dti.gov.uk and www.dwp.gov.uk or your local Jobcentre Plus office can help you with more information.

at a glance

❉ You are entitled to maternity leave and time off for antenatal care.

❉ Your employer cannot discriminate against you because you are pregnant.

❉ You are entitled to a workplace risk assessment once you have told your employer that you're pregnant. This is to ensure that where you work is safe for you and your baby.

❉ You must tell your employer:

– that you are pregnant

– the week your baby is expected to be born

– when you want your maternity leave to start.

Paternity leave

Two weeks paid paternity leave is now on offer for fathers. Statutory paternity pay (SPP) will be paid at a flat rate per week for two weeks (or 90% of average weekly earnings if this is less). The rate of statutory paternity pay is revised every April. Check with your Inland Revenue office for the current rate. Paternity leave can be taken from the date of the birth or up to eight weeks from the birth. To qualify for SPP, the father will need to have worked for his employer for 26 weeks by the 26th week of pregnancy and earn more than the lower earnings limit. He must also give his employer notice of the date on which he wants to start paternity leave by the 26th week of the pregnancy.

Child benefit

This is payable from the date the baby is born. It comes from the Benefits Agency. This is a regular payment made to anyone raising a child, it is not affected by income or savings and most people with a child qualify for it. It can be paid directly into your bank or savings account or through a Post Office or National Savings account that accepts Direct Payment. There is a form for child benefit in the bounty pack handed out by the hospital after your child is born. The form is also available online, visit **www.hmrc.gov.uk/childbenefit** or phone **0845 302 1444**.

Sure Start maternity grant

This is a lump sum grant for expectant mothers on income support, income-based job seekers allowance, parent credit or child tax credit. You do not have to pay back any of this money. To qualify, you must send in a certificate signed by an approved health professional confirming that you are under their care or have asked their advice because of having a baby. Claim your grant using form SF100 Sure Start which you can get from your local Jobcentre Plus office. You can claim at any time from the 29th week of pregnancy until your child is three months old.

For more information visit **www.newdeal.gov.uk** or **www.jobcentreplus.gov.uk**

Child trust fund

Every child receives money from the government. This money is for a child trust fund account – funds that are intended to build up and be cashed in when the child reaches 18. They cannot be touched until then. Family and friends can pay in up to £1,200 each year to boost the fund. All income and capital growth will be free from tax and the government makes another payment when your child is seven years old. For more information see **www.childtrustfund.gov.uk**

Childcare vouchers

From April 2005, your employer has been allowed to give pay in the form of vouchers for child care. No tax or national insurance will be taken off the first £55 a week or £243 per month of this allowance. See **www.hmrc.gov.uk/childcare** for more details.

Healthy Start

You will qualify for Healthy Start if you are pregnant and you or your family receive income support, income-based Jobseeker's Allowance or child tax credit (but not working tax credit) with an income below £16,190 a year. All pregnant women under the age of 18 also qualify, whether or not they are on benefits. Once accepted on to the scheme, pregnant women and families receive a set of vouchers through the post every four weeks. These vouchers can be exchanged for any combination of milk, fresh fruit, fresh vegetables, vitamins and infant formula milk in registered shops. For more information visit the Healthy Start website **www.healthystart.nhs.uk** or call the Healthy Start helpline on **0845 607 6823**.

Single parents

One Parent Families Scotland run a telephone helpline for single parents and pregnant women which, among other things, gives advice and support on benefits, call **0808 801 0323**.

The most up-to-date information on benefits can be found at **www.direct.gov.uk**

week 26-27

You may find your ankles and fingers swelling – sit with your feet up whenever you can.

With week 27 you are officially into your third trimester – late pregnancy. Or on the home stretch if you want to call it that!

Your baby's chances of surviving outside the uterus are growing by the week.

She is gaining fat and muscle and looks a little less skinny now.

She may begin to open and close her eyes.

You are walking differently because your centre of gravity has changed.

Tax credits

You may also be eligible for child tax and working tax credit. Child tax credit is a payment created to support families or individuals with at least one child or young person who they are responsible for. For more information please visit **www.taxcredits.direct.gov.uk** or call **0845 300 3900**.

Free dental care and free prescriptions

You are entitled to free prescriptions and free NHS dental treatment during your pregnancy and for the first year after giving birth.

Premature birth or preterm babies

Some babies arrive earlier than expected or are too sick to cope on their own. If this happens to your baby, you may not be able to take her home with you. Instead, your baby might need the special care of the neonatal (new born) unit or children's hospital.

When your baby arrives early

Preterm labour is generally defined as labour beginning before the 37th week of pregnancy. Over the last few years, babies born early have had a greater chance of surviving and developing without any long-term problems. The outlook for a preterm baby is affected by several things:

O The number of weeks you are pregnant. The older the baby is the better the chances of survival.

O The baby's size. Bigger babies usually have a better chance of survival, as long as they are healthy in other ways.

O Whether the baby has any birth abnormality.

O The availability of specialist care.

Why are some babies born early?

It's not always known why women go into labour early. Some possible reasons include:

- infection in the mother

- conditions such as pre-eclampsia

- more than one baby – most twins and triplets are born before 38 weeks, and many sooner than this – the uterus starts to contract when it is overstretched

- weakness in the cervix.

If your labour starts early, you will either realise the membranes have ruptured (your waters will 'break') or you will start to feel contractions. If you suspect you are in labour, or if you are bleeding, call the hospital straight away.

It may be possible to slow down or even stop your labour. Drugs that stop you having contractions may give your baby more time in the uterus. You may also be given treatment to prevent your baby being born with respiratory distress syndrome, a condition that seriously affects breathing.

Occasionally, a mother may be told that she needs to have her labour induced (started early) because she has a condition that threatens her health or her baby's health if the pregnancy continues. Sometimes the baby may have a better chance of survival outside the uterus (see page 85 for more information on induction).

Bliss is an organisation which provides vital support and care to premature and sick babies across the UK. Phone their free helpline on 0500 618140.

week 28

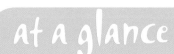

She can turn her head towards a bright continuous light.

Her skin is beginning to plump up and look more baby-like now.

Her brain is developing at a great pace.

You may have more tests about now (*see pages 36–40*).

As well as swollen ankles you may develop leg cramps – try not to stand for long periods and drink plenty of water.

You may start feeling so-called Braxton Hicks or practice contractions (*see below for more information*).

(*see What to look for, page 88*).

at a glance

✳ Babies born early have a much better chance of surviving and developing normally than even a few years ago.

✳ It's not always known why some women go into labour early.

✳ If you suspect you are in labour or if you are bleeding, call the hospital immediately (*see What to look for, page 88*).

Braxton Hicks

Braxton Hicks contractions are sporadic uterine contractions.

What do Braxton Hicks feel like?

You may feel your abdomen tightening for about 30 seconds, several times a day, from week 28 onwards. This can be easy to mistake for labour. You will feel your abdomen harden and, if you are in the bath for example, you will see it remain tense for several seconds. Unlike labour contractions Braxton Hicks contractions don't increase in length, intensity or frequency and they are not painful. They tend to be short and come and go intermittently. Time them; this will help you decide if it is the real thing or not.

Are you in labour?

If you are less than 37 weeks pregnant and you're having more than four contractions in an hour as well as other signs of preterm labour, contact your midwife for advice.

Getting ready for parenthood

Parenthood is a life-changing event and it brings with it some big changes. There are lots of things to think about and prepare for – not just stocking up on nappies. The good news is that the most important thing your baby will need is you.

Equipment you will need

Very young babies don't need very much at all – most equipment isn't needed until they're a few months old or have reached a certain size.

The basics to begin with are:

- clothes
- nappies
- somewhere warm and clean to sleep
- something to ride or be carried in like a pram or pushchair with a 'lie-back' position, or a sling
- bedding
- bottles and sterilising equipment for formula fed babies *(see pages 128–131)*
- car safety seat *(see page 133)*.

You may also choose to have some of the following, but these aren't essential:

- a baby bath – not essential as your baby can use the big bath or even a clean washing-up bowl at first
- a crib or Moses basket – easier to move around than the 'big' cot but soon outgrown
- a changing mat or table.

Balancing saving money with safety

Buying or borrowing second-hand equipment is a good idea only when you know its full history. When buying a second-hand cot or Moses basket make sure you buy a new mattress that fits properly. Second-hand clothing or shared/borrowed clothing is a good way to save money. *(See **Thinking about safety** 82–83)*.

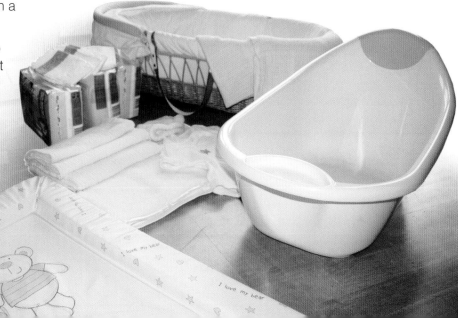

week 29-30

Your baby is about 38.5 cm (a little more than 15 inches) from head to toe.

She's making breathing movements more regularly — she may surprise you if she has the hiccups.

You may be a little forgetful (well, pregnancy is a good excuse!) You could also be a bit clumsier than usual.

Your baby is getting on for 1.5 kilos (about 2½ lbs). She is growing fast.

Good posture can help relieve the strain on your back as can gentle massage.

You may find it hard to sleep — try sleeping with a cushion between your knees or at your side to make yourself comfortable.

The lanugo (fine hair covering your baby's body) may be starting to fall out.

Preparing for parenthood and your emotions

You've probably just become used to some of the new emotions of being pregnant and expecting a baby. Now you may start to focus on what it will be like after she arrives and you become a fully-fledged mum. You may be excited or nervous, or both.

What you may be worried about

If you already have a child or children you may wonder how the new baby will fit into your family and how her brothers or sisters will react. If this is your first baby you may wonder how you'll cope with the responsibility and change. Both you and your partner may worry about how it will affect your work and social life and whether you will do a good job.

It's perfectly natural to have fears and anxieties about parenthood. Your partner probably has them too. Talking about it can help and your midwife and antenatal classes should be able to reassure you.

At a glance

✳ Think safety! Do not use second-hand equipment unless you know its history and, in the case of car seats for example, make sure you have the manufacturer's instructions.

✳ Don't go overboard— there are only a few essentials that you absolutely have to have.

✳ Help is available for mums-to-be with low incomes.

✳ You don't have to buy everything at once.

Planning for the birth

You will have lots of questions about the birth, from where it will take place to what exactly happens. You'll also need to make some decisions and there is plenty of information and support to help you.

What sort of birth is right for you?

Your midwife may ask you during pregnancy if you would like to make a birth plan. This means that your choices are written down, after a full discussion covering all the information you need to make your choice.

The birth plan then goes into your notes, with a copy for you to keep. Your choices are important guidelines and reminders, but you can still change your mind.

If you are confused about anything or have concerns, talk to your midwife or antenatal teacher.

Making a birth plan

Things to consider for your birth plan are:

- whether you want to be free to move into different positions during labour and delivery

- how you want your baby's heart rate to be monitored

- whether you want an actively managed or 'physiological' third stage of labour *(see page 104)*

- how you feel about induction and acceleration of labour

- that vitamin K will be given to your baby after she is delivered unless you make a decision otherwise *(see page 59).*

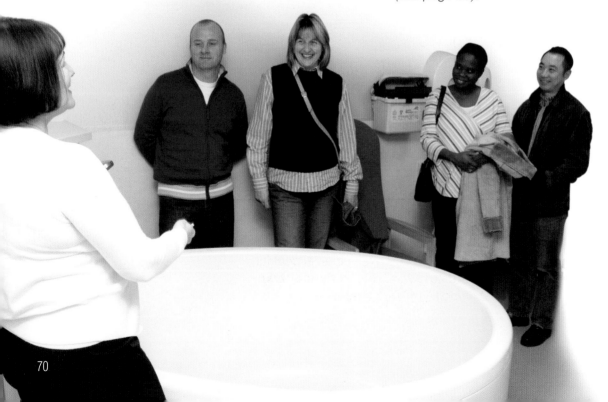

week 31-32

You may notice stretch marks if you haven't already.

You may notice your baby moving less. Don't worry – she's just running out of space.

Even when you feel a bit breathless your baby is getting all the oxygen she needs from the placenta.

She can close her eyes in response to bright light outside your abdomen.

Your baby is about 42 cm (16½ inches) from head to toe.

You may be panicking about how much you still have to do.

Her lungs are formed and maturing and she is still putting on weight.

There's some evidence that your baby dreams while she's asleep.

You may be getting indigestion because of pressure from your baby on your stomach.

Who will be with you at the birth?

Who would you like to give you support and encouragement when you're in labour? Your partner may be the obvious choice, if you have one, but it doesn't have to be. It can be a friend or your mum.

There is some evidence that having another person with you, instead of (or as well as) your partner, is helpful and can shorten your labour. Some women have a close friend, a relative or their antenatal teacher.

It's a good idea to discuss your birth plan with your partner and whoever else will be with you at the birth. If they know what you expect and what your decisions are they'll be able to give you better support.

Water birth

You can discuss the possibility of delivering your baby in the water with the midwife/midwives who will be caring for you (if you plan a home birth) or with the antenatal clinic and the labour ward midwife (if you plan to give birth in hospital).

If you would like to stay in the water for a long time, it's better to use a large pool giving you plenty of room in which to change positions. The midwife can examine you in the pool if necessary, and help deliver your baby. The water needs to be kept warm. Some hospitals have a birthing pool or a large bath they use for labour. You can hire a special pool for use at home or in units where they are not available (see **Further help** page 206). Discuss what's available locally with your midwife.

At a glance

❋ Who will be your birth companion(s)?

❋ Do you want to use a birth pool or bath?

❋ Have you considered how you will cope with pain during labour?

Labouring in water can help you relax, and women often report that it helps lessen the pain of contractions. More women use the pool for labour than actually give birth to their baby in it.

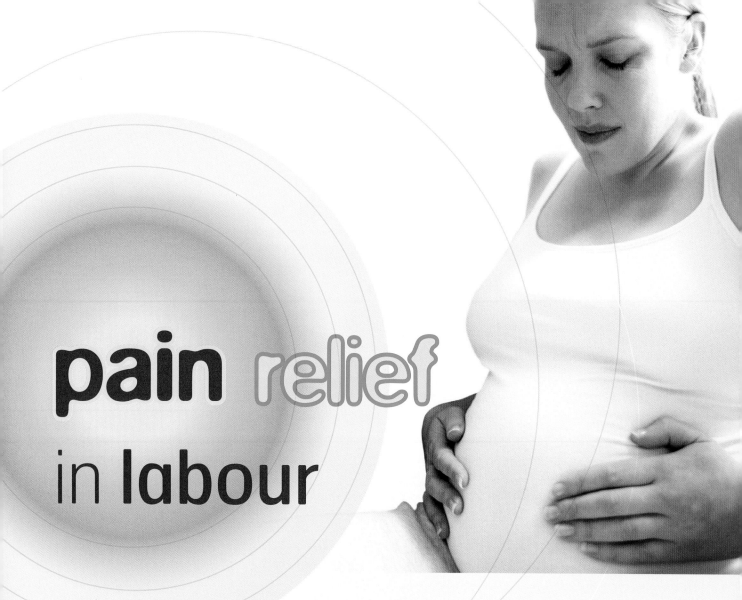

pain relief
in labour

Thinking about pain relief beforehand will give you a chance to find out what is available and how it will affect you and your baby. Your midwife will tell you what's available. You'll be able to talk about your choices in antenatal classes too *(see page 44)*.

You may wish to use self-help forms of pain relief or to have pain-relieving drugs of some type.

There are different options and, depending on where you will give birth, different choices may be available to you. Most women use breathing and relaxation techniques whether or not they choose to have pain-relieving drugs.

It's important to think about how you want to cope with the pain before labour begins.

non-chemical pain relief

There are different forms of pain relief aside from pain-relieving drugs. The primary one is breathing and relaxation techniques but birthing pools and lying in water are also considered non-chemical ways of helping you cope with the pain. Other methods of non-drug pain relief are things like TENS-machine, homeopathy, hypnosis, acupuncture or acupressure. You will need to see a specialised practitioner if you are interested in these methods.

Most antenatal classes teach breathing awareness as a way of coping with the pain of contractions. The emphasis is on breathing as a way of relaxation, which helps you cope with the pain.

Relaxation doesn't take away pain, but it can prevent pain becoming stronger, because tension increases pain levels. The main aim is to help you cope with the pain and not be overwhelmed by it. Then you will be fully conscious and in as much control of your labour as you want to be. Research shows that when women are relaxed they release the body's own, hormone-like, pain relievers – endorphins.

Effects

Some women want to avoid drugs in labour, as all drug-based pain relief has some disadvantages to mother or baby or both. You may want to rely on yourself, with the support and encouragement of those around you. There are no disadvantages to breathing and relaxation, but sometimes it may not work if your labour is very long or complicated or is just too painful for you.

epidural anaesthesia

An epidural refers to a pain relieving drug which is injected into the epidural space around your spinal nerves. This stops sensation in your lower body and relieves pain; it may cause your lower body to feel numb. It does not cause you to lose consciousness.

How it works

You may be asked to curl up on your side while the anaesthetist inserts the epidural, or you may be able to sit up while leaning forward over a pillow. A fine plastic tube – an epidural catheter – will remain in your back so that more pain-relieving drugs can be given as needed. You will be given a drip so that fluids and intravenous medicines can be given if needed (low blood pressure can be a side-effect of the epidural).

It is likely that your baby's heartbeat will need to be continually monitored.

Effects

The aim of the epidural is to relieve the pain of labour while still allowing you to move around the bed and push effectively at delivery. Your legs might feel numb or heavy which can make it harder to push. The numbness can last up to a few hours after the delivery. Assisted delivery with forceps or ventouse (see page 100) may be more common. This may be because you are more likely to ask for an epidural if you are having a long or difficult labour.

Anaesthetic drugs can be delivered through the epidural catheter to allow an assisted delivery or even a Caesarean section, if needed.

Epidural may not be available at every unit.

Occasionally you may have a bad headache for some days after the birth. Mild itching is also possible with some pain relieving drugs. You may also experience some tenderness around the epidural insertion but epidurals have been shown not to cause long-term backache.

As an epidural delivers opiates into your and your baby's system, your baby is likely to be sleepy and may not take to feeding right away. You'll be given extra support to help you through this.

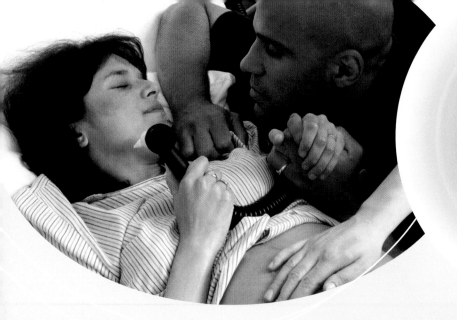

At home, the midwife can give you gas and air. In hospital, all forms of pain relief are available, although in some units epidurals may not be.

gas and air

Entonox and Equanox are brand names for a mix of gas and air (50% nitrous oxide and 50% oxygen) that can be used to help you through the pain of contractions. This is usually referred to simply as 'gas' or 'gas and air'. This form of pain relief is available in hospital and at home births.

How it works

The gas comes with a tube and a mask or mouthpiece that you can breathe through when you need it – usually at the start of a contraction. It starts to work within about 15–20 seconds after first breathing in. You can keep breathing in and as you start to feel light headed and drowsy your hand holding the mouthpiece will drop away. It can take the 'edge' off the peak of pain and the relief should last to the end of the contraction. The pain relief does not last very long and for it to work effectively you need to begin breathing it at the very start of the contraction so it builds up by the time you are at the peak of it.

Effects

Because you become drowsy when inhaling the gas and you naturally stop breathing it in there is no danger of taking too much. Your body expels the gas quickly. It can make some people nauseous. Using gas does not prevent you from using other pain relief.

Babies do not appear to be affected as very little gas reaches them.

morphine and opiate drugs

Drugs that are related to morphine are commonly given in labour and can be used at home too. The use of opiates at a home birth is strongly discouraged because they may cause breathing difficulties for the baby and these can be better dealt with at hospital. They are given by injection and the dose can be varied.

Effects

Most morphine and opiate drugs take around 15 minutes to work and last for two to four hours. You may feel sleepy and slightly 'out of it', as if the pain is there but you're not experiencing it. Some women feel this distancing effect as being out of control. Some feel sick with these drugs and an anti-sickness medicine is usually given at the same time.

All opiates can affect the baby's breathing at birth. The baby may be sleepier and less interested in feeding for two or three days afterwards. If your baby's breathing is poor because of the opiates, a drug can be given to treat this. This effect on breathing is more likely if the injection is given too close to the birth, and you may be advised not to have it for this reason. If opiates are given four or more hours before birth, the effects have a better chance of wearing off in the mother. The effects will remain in the baby for longer, say up to 48 hours, after birth.

You should discuss pain relief with your midwife.

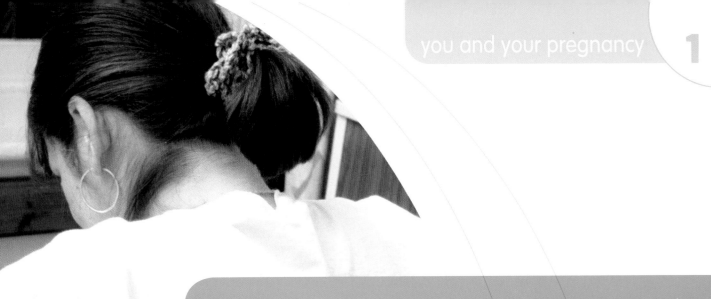

TENS (transcutaneous electrical nerve stimulation)

TENS (transcutaneous electrical nerve stimulation) is a form of pain relief provided by a small box wired to electrodes which fix on your skin, and which give out a slight electrical charge. It can be effective in relieving pain, and it is safe for you and does not affect your baby. If you want to use this, ask your midwife where you can hire or borrow a TENS machine so that you can start to use it as soon as labour begins.

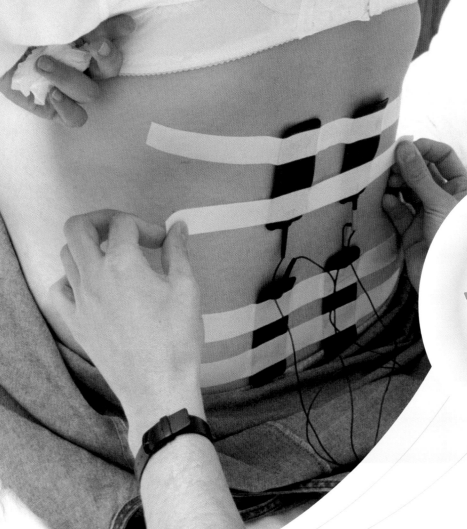

It's up to you what sort of pain relief you want – whether it is natural or some form of drug – and you can change your mind if you want to.

Getting organised: what to pack

As you get closer to your due date there are lots of things to arrange. It makes sense to have a bag packed and ready to go. You'll probably want to pack two bags, one with things you want for the actual labour and one with everything you'll need afterwards – including something for your new baby to wear going home!

Bag one (labour)

- ✓ mineral water spray or a plant spray with a fine nozzle – put it in a fridge (if possible) to keep it cool
- ✓ two facecloths for cooling your face and skin
- ✓ music player
- ○ unscented oil or a light body lotion for massage
- ✓ thermal pack (the sort you can heat in a microwave for taking with you on cold outings – it stays warm for hours); it can be wrapped in a towel and used as a warm compress to relieve aches in the back or in the legs
- ✓ old nightdress (front opening for easy breastfeeding) or old T-shirt
- ✓ dressing-gown (robe) and sandals or slippers
- ✓ hairbrush
- ✓ hair bands for long hair
- ✓ wash bag with toiletries
- ✓ toothbrush and toothpaste
- ✓ phone card/coins
- ✓ camera
- ○ drinks and snacks for you and your partner.

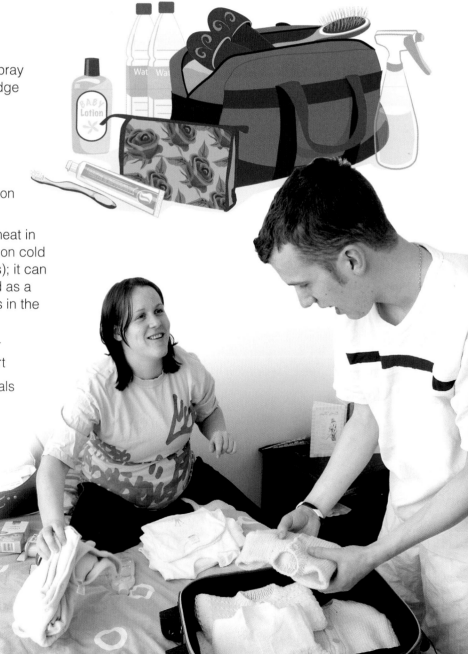

week 33-34

Your baby's lungs are now fully developed.

Your tummy button may be sticking out.

Your breasts may start to leak colostrum in preparation for breastfeeding. This doesn't happen to everyone.

Your baby may be lying head down in preparation for being born.

Her skin is getting smoother.

She can do all sorts of baby things such as suck and grab – not that there's much in there to get hold of.

The puffiness may be getting worse – if your face is swelling too, check with your midwife or GP (see page 79).

Drinking plenty of water can help with fluid retention.

Resting with your feet up will help deal with varicose veins.

Bag two (after the birth)

- ☑ two nightdresses (front opening for easy breastfeeding)
- ○ easy to wear dayclothes (like a jogging suit – again front opening for easy breastfeeding)
- ☑ underwear, including large, close-fitting pants (to hold maternity pads), and nursing bras – you may find disposable pants useful for the first few days
- ☑ towels
- ☑ maternity pads or night-time sanitary pads
- ☑ breast pads

- ○ tissues
- ☑ phone card/coins
- ○ unscented toiletries and cosmetics
- ☑ nappies for baby
- ☑ vests and sleep suits
- ○ cotton wool balls and nappy cream
- ○ fruit juice/mineral water
- ○ healthy snacks.

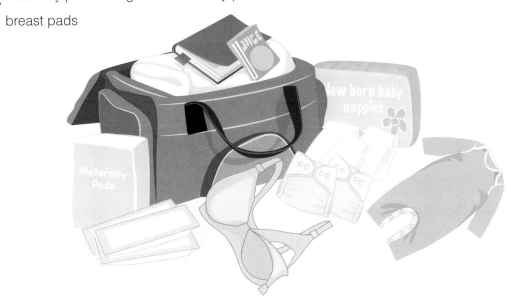

Your baby's position

Your baby's position or 'presentation' refers to which part of the baby's body will be born first. Although most babies are born head first sometimes they are in breech presentation. Some babies who come head first are in the posterior position.

Breech position

This means your baby is lying head up in the uterus. Her bottom (or, occasionally her foot) is probably the part that will be born first – the 'presenting' part. Babies may lie with their legs bent at the knees, almost cross-legged, or with their knees pointing up towards the face – this is known as 'frank breech'.

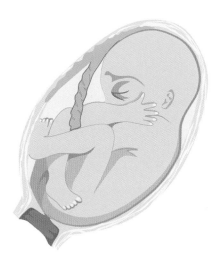

How common is breech?

At 30 weeks of pregnancy, about 20% of babies are in the breech position. By the end of pregnancy only about 3% are breech. Many babies move into a head-down (vertex) position by themselves.

Babies who are still breech by about 37 weeks of pregnancy may not turn by themselves. Some doctors try to turn them by 'external cephalic version' (ECV). ECV is not usually done before 37 weeks or the end of term. If it is needed your midwife will explain this procedure to you and answer any questions you may have.

Delivering a breech baby

Almost all doctors prefer to deliver breech babies by Caesarean section as research shows this is less likely to harm the baby. If your baby is expected to be born breech some options for where to give birth may not be available to you – you will not be able to have a home birth for example. You can talk about this with your midwife.

Posterior position

The posterior position refers to when your baby's back is lying against your back. It doesn't matter earlier on but once you are ready to go into labour your baby has to turn all the way around to the front. While in the posterior position your baby's head presses against your sacrum (your lower back) and can cause backache which can be worse in labour.

What you can do

There are some things you can do before your baby is born which may help your baby turn. From about 36 weeks you can try leaning forward whenever you can. This may help your baby to turn so that her back is toward your front, before her head becomes engaged in your pelvis in preparation for the birth.

week 35
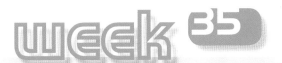

Try to rest as much as you can – you'll be tired and there won't be much time for rest after the birth!

Take some gentle exercise – for example a walk or a swim. It'll help you relax and make it easier to sleep.

Your baby's toenails and fingernails could almost do with a trim!

If you haven't thought of a name yet, visit your library to borrow a book on baby names.

She weighs around 2.3 kg (a little more than 5 lbs) and is still gaining!

Your feet are bigger – slip-on shoes are easier to get on and off.

pre-eclampsia

This condition occurs only in pregnancy and affects 1 in every 10 pregnancies. Most cases are mild, but some (about one first pregnancy in every 100) are dangerous for the baby and the mother.

If you have severe pre-eclampsia or eclampsia, your labour may be induced, even though this may mean a preterm delivery.

The condition is called 'pre' (before) eclampsia because, if it is not treated or is treated too late, it can develop into eclampsia, a rare but serious complication with seizures or fits. However, eclampsia is not the only serious complication of pre-eclampsia; you may also develop problems with your liver, lungs, kidneys, brain or blood-clotting system.

Some of the signs and symptoms of pre-eclampsia are:

- rising blood pressure in mid to late pregnancy

- protein in the urine

In serious cases of pre-eclampsia, you may feel very unwell. You may vomit, have a bad headache and visual disturbances, and severe pain just below the ribs. Report these symptoms to your midwife urgently.

- severe oedema (swelling) due to fluid retention in the ankles, fingers or face

- headaches/visual disturbances

- severe pain just below the ribs

- poor growth of the baby.

Routine antenatal checking of your blood pressure and your urine is done mainly to watch out for pre-eclampsia.

The causes of pre-eclampsia and high blood pressure are not fully understood, and the links between the main signs are still very unclear. If you have any of the signs or any concerns speak to your midwife immediately.

Caesarean births

You may know that you need a Caesarean birth before you go into labour. In some cases a decision has to be made to have a Caesarean birth while you are in labour.

What is a Caesarean birth?

A Caesarean birth means your baby is born by an operation. The obstetrician makes an opening in your abdomen and then the uterus. In your notes, you may see it as LSCS or LUSCS, which is the abbreviation for lower segment Caesarean section or lower uterine segment Caesarean section, or simply as CS (Caesarean section).

Why it's done

A Caesarean section may be planned in advance. This is called an 'elective section'. Your appointment will probably be before the date your baby is due (your expected date of delivery) so you won't go into labour before the operation.

You may go into labour and expect to give birth vaginally, but then find you need a Caesarean section. This is called an emergency Caesarean section, although often it isn't as dramatic or last-minute as the name suggests.

Anaesthesia and Caesarean section

If you have a Caesarean section, you will need total pain relief. Some women have a general anaesthetic, which works instantly and means you are unconscious during the operation. Most women have an epidural or spinal anaesthetic. This completely numbs you from just below the breasts downwards, but allows you to remain fully awake and aware of everything except the pain.

It takes time to recover from the effects of a general anaesthetic and there are more risks to the mother's health, so epidural or spinal anaesthesia will usually be given. In some units, doctors administer a combined spinal and epidural which allows a top-up of anaesthetic when necessary. This type of anaesthesia takes effect in about 15 minutes. You are more likely to need a general anaesthetic for an emergency Caesarean section if the baby is in distress and the doctor has to get her out as quickly as possible. You will receive help and support to make sure you are able to breastfeed comfortably after a Caesarean section if you wish.

What happens next

The obstetrician first makes a cut at the base of your abdomen and then through the uterus, in a line called a bikini incision.

You may feel some tugging when the baby is lifted out, sometimes by hand, sometimes with a pair of forceps. The baby's umbilical cord is clamped and cut, and then she will be quickly checked over. If all is well you will be given your baby to hold as soon as possible. The placenta and membranes are delivered next, and then your uterus and abdomen are stitched. It only takes about ten minutes to deliver the baby and about 30 minutes to stitch you afterwards.

Why you may need an elective Caesarean section

- You have a very low-lying placenta (called placenta praevia) which blocks your baby's way out.

- Multiple pregnancy – for some twins and almost always for triplets or more.

- Other complications, such as previous vaginal surgery.

- Malpresentation – your baby is in a position which makes vaginal birth difficult or impossible.

week 36

You baby probably weighs about 2.7 kg (about 6 lbs).

She is still moving, but movement is reduced (there's not much room in there).

You should feel movements each day, however small.

Her head may be 'engaged' – which means the widest part of the head has passed below the pelvic brim (known as 'engagement').

Your antenatal appointments will probably be more regular now.

Your bump is getting lower – called lightening – as your baby is preparing to be born.

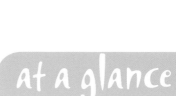

at a glance

✻ Normal vaginal delivery is natural and usually safer, but isn't always possible.

✻ Around a quarter of babies are born via Caesarean section.

✻ It's a major operation and you may take some time to recover.

✻ You may know in advance that you will have a Caesarean section (known as 'elective') or it may be unplanned ('emergency').

Why you may need an emergency Caesarean section

- Eclampsia or severe pre-eclampsia in the mother *(see page 79)* which means the baby should be delivered urgently.

- Onset of severe illness, such as kidney disease, or very high blood pressure.

- Your baby is suffering from fetal distress (lack of oxygen) and labour hasn't gone far enough for a forceps or a ventouse delivery *(see page 100)* to be carried out safely.

- Your baby's head is too big for your pelvis (disproportion), or your pelvic shape or size won't allow the baby to be born without major difficulty or risk.

- Lack of progress in labour, your contractions are weak and your cervix doesn't dilate.

Thinking about safety

Your baby relies on you to keep her safe. Of course you'll have to take more steps to improve your home's safety once she can move for herself *(see page 186)*. But there are things you can do before you get her home.

Safety for you and your baby

○ Have your gas appliances or gas or oil heating checked. Consider fitting carbon monoxide detectors.

○ Keep the stairs clear of clutter – you could easily trip while carrying the baby or while pregnant.

○ Keep a well-stocked first-aid kit in the kitchen or bathroom.

○ Get into the habit of putting medicines, vitamin tablets and other dangerous substances such as both oils and cleaning materials out of reach or locked away.

○ Write a list of important numbers (such as GP, hospital, work) by the phone, or somewhere else easy to find, to use in an emergency – why not write them in the front of this book?

○ Fit fireguards on all fires.

○ Know how you and your family can leave the house safely and quickly if there's a fire. Plan your escape and make sure the whole family knows what to do and practise it.

○ Place non-slip mats under rugs or unfitted carpet.

○ Some local authorities have home safety officers – you can get the number in the telephone book. Your health visitor/public health nurse should also be able to advise on home safety.

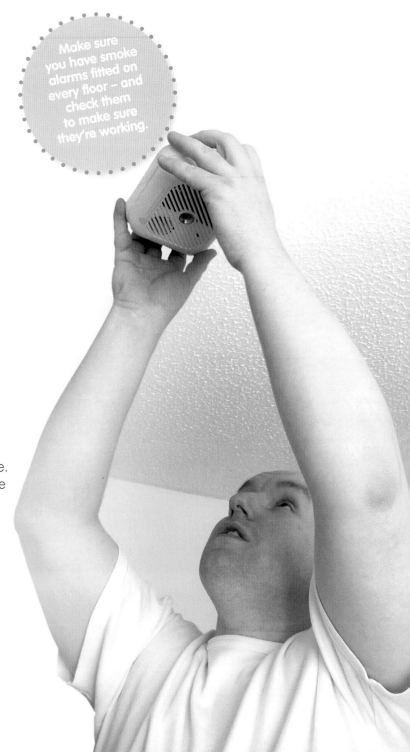

Make sure you have smoke alarms fitted on every floor – and check them to make sure they're working.

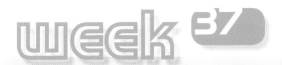

week 37

Your baby's putting on weight at about half an ounce (14 g) a day.

Take plenty of rest – labour and childbirth will take it out of you!

You should already have your bags packed.

You'll be getting curious about what she will look like.

Safety in the car

You must have a car seat for your baby if you plan to take her in a car, even for a short trip or in a taxi. Some taxi firms will provide car seats on request but you will need to check with them beforehand. Some hospitals will not allow parents to leave in a car after the birth without demonstrating that they have an infant carrier so it's important to plan this ahead of time. Never carry your baby on your lap.

When it comes to choosing a car seat you'll need to decide between a rear-facing seat and combination seat which can be turned once your baby is bigger. It is particularly important that you know how to fit the seat properly in the car. If you are buying an infant carrier ask for a demonstration from the sales assistant or see *The Good Egg Guide to In-car Child Safety*, available from some health boards and online at **www.protectchild.co.uk**

Babies and young children should never be left alone inside a vehicle, even when the engine is turned off. Never leave the keys in the ignition when you get out of the car.

at a glance

✳ It's never too early to make your home safer.

✳ Make sure you have a working smoke alarm.

✳ Practise fitting your carseat into your car.

✳ Your local fire and rescue service will provide free advice about fitting fire alarms. They may even supply them.

✳ See *The Scottish Good Egg Guide to Keeping Your Child Safe at Home* for more tips visit www.protectchild.co.uk

general safety advice

It's worth thinking about these things now so that they're second nature when your baby comes home.

○ Never, ever shake a baby – it can cause brain damage and even be fatal.

○ Don't have a hot drink while holding a baby as it could spill and cause scalding – and don't let visitors do it either. Hot drinks are the cause of most scalding injuries with babies.

○ Bear in mind that other people's houses may not be 'baby-proofed'.

When travelling with your baby, it's illegal not to have a properly fitted car seat in a car you own or someone else's.

Last-minute things to think about

So the big day's almost arrived. You're probably excited and a bit nervous. Take some time to get yourself organised so you're not in a rush at the last minute.

You may find this checklist useful:

○ Are all your emergency numbers (such as your labour ward, midwife, taxi) to hand?

○ Do you have the numbers of everyone you will wish to notify after the birth?

○ Is your bag packed? *(See pages 76–77).*

○ Do you have your birth plan? *(See page 70).*

○ Do you have your maternity notes?

○ Have you thought about the options for pain relief during labour? *(See pages 72–75).*

○ Can you easily get hold of your partner or whoever you want to be with you when you give birth?

○ Is there someone else on hand in case you can't get in touch with them?

○ If you have young children, have you made arrangements for their care during the labour and birth?

○ Do you have a car seat suitable for the baby and car – and have you practised fitting it? *(See page 133).*

○ Is your home safe for the baby? *(See pages 82–83).*

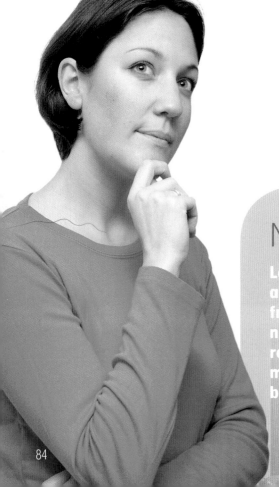

Mobile phones and texting

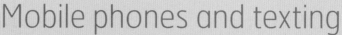

Lots of couples find that texting the good news is a quick and convenient way of letting family and friends know so it's a good idea to have everyone's numbers stored in your phone in advance. But remember to check your hospital's policy on using mobile phones as you may have to go outside the building before switching it on.

week 38
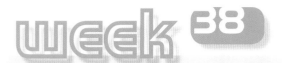

Although week 40 is your due date, remember that most babies are either late or early.

Your Braxton Hicks contractions could be more frequent and stronger.

Taking a gentle walk may ease some of your aches and pains.

Your baby is making movements every day. If she isn't, inform your midwife straight away.

Your baby is fully developed and ready to go – at her own pace, that is.

She's still covered in vernix but the lanugo has gone.

Your due date

It's a rare baby that turns up on the exact due date, which means most will be either early or late.

Late babies

It's still a mystery why some babies are late. In some cases, it may be that the due date has simply been wrong. Not that that's much help to you and your partner as you sit there day after day wondering if this will be the one when it happens!

Provided the pregnancy has developed normally, there's probably no need for doctors to intervene until you reach 42 weeks, although different units may have different policies. After this, there is a higher risk of problems at the birth.

Inducing labour

It is sometimes necessary to start labour artificially. This is known as induction of labour. If this is necessary your midwife will advise you.

> I'm so excited but at the same time really nervous. I can't wait to meet my new baby.
>
> *Jane, Stirling*

at a glance

✣ Most babies will be either early or late.

✣ Medical staff may suggest helping the baby along (inducing) at 42 weeks.

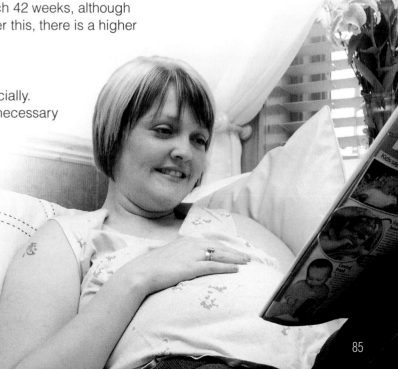

labour and birth

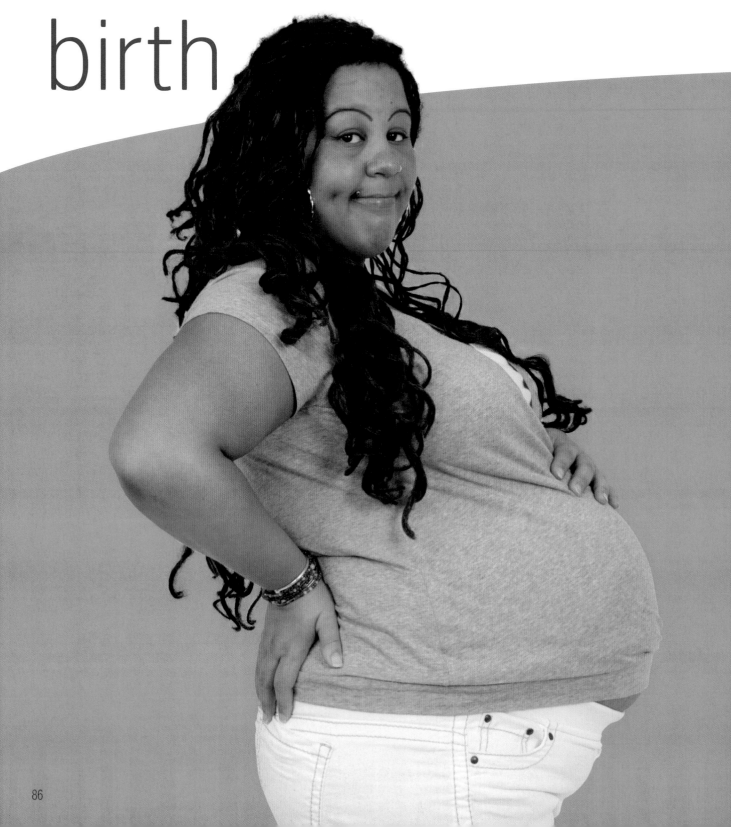

Section 2

What to **look for**

Labour can start very quickly or it can seem to take ages. Sometimes it can start without you realising it. The start of the first stage is often slow and it may take a while to establish that you are actually in labour. Once you are well dilated, your contractions are longer and stronger and your labour progresses more quickly.

There are obvious signs of labour

The 'show': this is the release of the mucus plug, which seals the opening of the cervix. In some women it comes out of the vagina as a single blob of pinkish jelly; in others it is a series of smaller pieces, and in others it can be reddish brown and blood tinged.

It is a sign that the cervix is beginning to stretch and soften a little, in preparation for labour. It may not mean you are actually in labour. It can be several days between the show and the start of labour proper, or just an hour or so, or anything in between.

The breaking of the waters: the amniotic sac is the bag of fluid surrounding the baby inside the uterus.

When the membranes break, or rupture, the fluid escapes. It can happen as a sudden gush of liquid down your legs. More usually though, it will start to trickle. There may be a risk of infection to the baby if the membranes rupture and labour doesn't start within a day or so. If the baby's head is not yet engaged, or if your baby is breech, a rush of waters may bring the cord with it. The cord could then become compressed which would be risky for your baby's oxygen supply. Telephone your midwife or the hospital if your waters break.

Contractions: these are the only sure signs of labour if they gradually come closer together and last longer than 40 seconds. You should feel them getting stronger, longer and more rhythmical, too.

false alarms

Sometimes women start to have contractions only for them to fade away. These can be deceptive, and make you think you are in labour. You go to hospital, only to find everything stops. If this happens to you, you may be examined, and may be disappointed that you are not very far on in your labour; maybe your cervix doesn't show that the contractions have had any effect at all. In this situation, you may be asked if you'd prefer to go home. This is sensible, unless you live a long way from the hospital. Don't feel embarrassed. This sort of false alarm happens all the time.

the **first stage**

Health professionals normally describe labour as being in three stages. The first stage is usually the longest and can last anything from one hour to 20 hours or even longer.

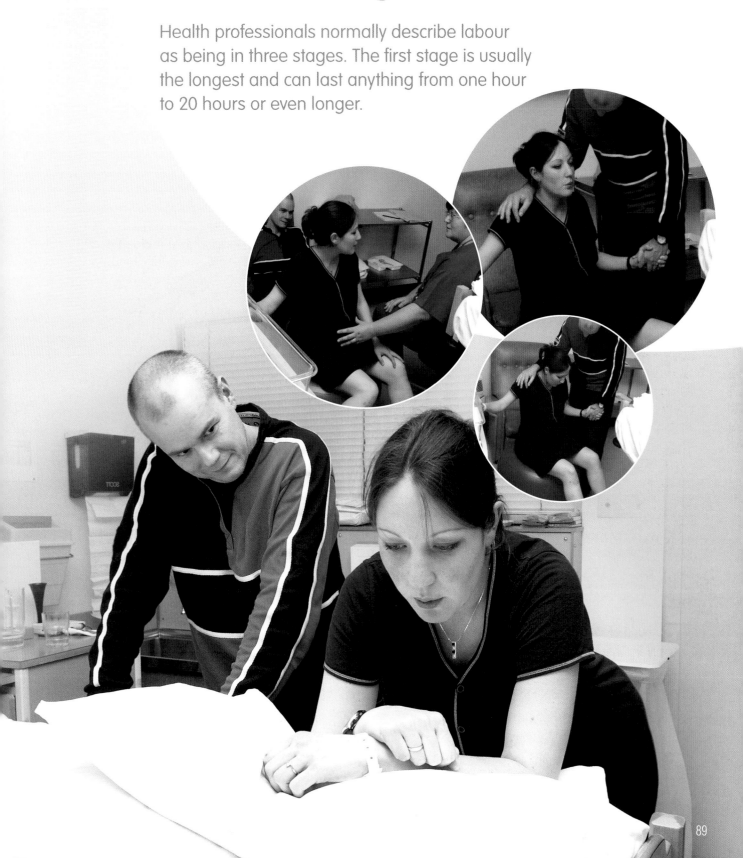

Early labour

We've all heard stories about people who have been in labour for many hours and others who had their babies within minutes. Most are somewhere in between. The important thing is that while they vary, they're all normal.

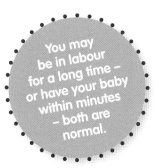

Starting out

It can be boring and frustrating waiting for things to pick up the pace, you may go to hospital only to find you are not very far along at all *(see page 88, **False alarms**)*. If you are not sure what to do, contact the maternity unit or your community midwife. You will describe your symptoms and be advised on whether you should do anything other than wait and see what happens. You may have a visit from a midwife who can examine you and help you decide the best place to be.

> I wasn't sure if I wanted my partner there when I gave birth but actually it was great, even in the early stages when there wasn't much happening – we probably talked more than we've done in ages. We've both been so busy preparing for the baby.
>
> *Gillian, Hamilton*

In the meantime try to relax by:

- taking deep relaxing breaths
- having a bath or shower
- having your partner give you a gentle massage
- using an ice pack or hot water bottle on your back if you are uncomfortable
- walking around
- eating a light snack and drinking plenty of water or fruit juice.

sex and labour

There is a widespread idea that sexual activity can start labour, when the baby is ready to be born. There may be some basis to this. Semen has natural prostaglandins (hormones) in it, and may stimulate the cervix to 'ripen' a little more.

Sexual stimulation in the woman releases hormones – oxytocins – which are released in labour, too. There's no evidence that any sexual activity starts labour too soon. If labour was about to begin anyway, then sex may help it a little.

How you may be feeling

It's normal to feel nervous about the birth, especially if it seems to be taking forever and you are scared about the pain. It's also quite normal to decide at this point that you'd like the baby to just stay in there – this isn't an option!

Try to keep the end goal in your mind. At the end of labour, you'll have your baby. That's what the past 40 or so weeks have been about and now it's nearly time.

Contractions are steps on the way to achieving that goal – bringing you closer to meeting your baby. And although they are usually painful, between each contraction you may not feel much pain at all.

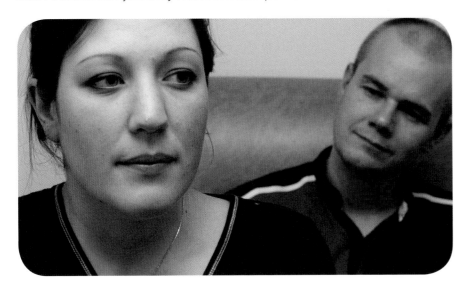

What are contractions?

Contractions are the regular tightening of the uterus, working to dilate the cervix (neck of the womb) and to push the baby down the birth canal. Contractions usually feel like a tightening sensation across your tummy and possibly into your back and thighs. Each one usually begins gently, builds up to a peak and then trails off. They may remind you of period pains (which are also contractions of the uterus), or feel much more painful. Women have different experiences with contractions, as the intensity can vary a lot.

At the start of the first stage, contractions may last about 40–50 seconds and you may get one every 10 minutes. By the end, each will last over a minute and there will be a gap of no more than a minute between them. Again, this can be different from woman to woman.

At this stage, contractions are opening the cervix to allow the baby to be born. This is called dilation. At the start, particularly if it's your first baby, labour often moves quite slowly. When you are five and six centimetres dilated the contractions get longer and stronger and labour progresses more quickly. This is called established labour.

at a glance

* There's no such thing as a 'typical' labour and birth – they're all different.

* The signs of labour can be difficult to recognise.

* Sometimes labour can seem to start then stop – if you're at all concerned, telephone your midwife or labour ward.

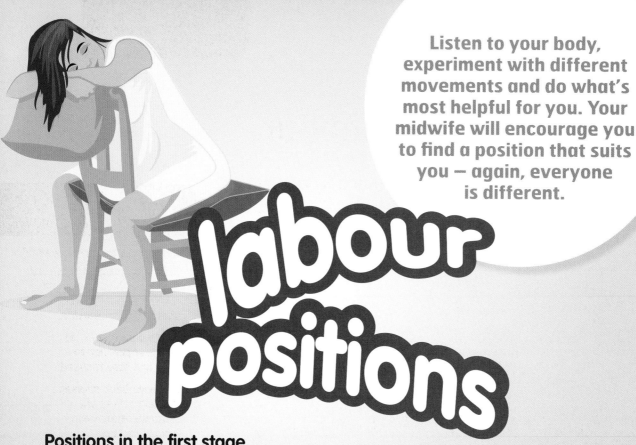

Listen to your body, experiment with different movements and do what's most helpful for you. Your midwife will encourage you to find a position that suits you – again, everyone is different.

labour positions

Positions in the first stage

Most women cope best with labour if they are not restricted in their movements. You may find different positions – supported standing, kneeling, sitting (either astride a chair or on a birthing ball) or anything else that helps – work best for you at different times.

Kneeling: you can rest by leaning forward between contractions.

Sitting: you can sit astride a chair and lean forward, rest on a cushion or pillow, or on a birthing ball or beanbag.

Birthing balls: you may find a birthing ball comfortable – this is a large inflatable ball which is used in some gyms. It allows you to rotate your pelvis and means you are sitting at a good angle for childbirth with your pelvis above your knees.

Supported standing or squatting: this allows your pelvis to open wide, and your baby to be born with the help of gravity. You will need support for your upper body to keep your balance. Your partner can support you by holding you from behind, under your arms, though they will need strength to take all your weight. Your knees must never be higher than your hips – this would put too much strain on your joints.

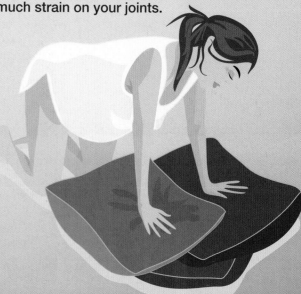

There's no right or wrong position. However, lying on your back is usually uncomfortable and makes it more difficult to get the baby through the pelvis, so it is not recommended. When women are encouraged to do what feels best, they hardly ever adopt this position.

Coping with early labour

Contractions are usually painful. You should have been given tips on how to cope at antenatal classes *(see page 44)* or by your midwife.

Ideally your partner or whoever is with you at the birth will also have an idea of what's going on and be there to support you. Partners can help by gently rubbing your back, holding your hand and generally being there to share the pain as well as the joy.

Breathing exercises can also help.

Your birthing partner can help you through your contractions by breathing with you if you find that helpful and letting you know when each contraction ends.

As you feel a contraction coming:

○ **Relax. Think especially about your shoulders, your face, your hands. Make sure they are relaxed.**

○ **Start to concentrate on your breathing, keeping it slow and relaxed. Focus on breathing out.**

○ **As the contraction gets stronger, think more carefully about the way you breathe and try to stay relaxed.**

○ **Sway and rock your pelvis; make any noises you find helpful.**

○ **Don't resist the contraction — it increases in intensity, reaches its height, then starts to fade.**

○ **As it goes, blow it away. It's gone. That contraction will never appear again, and it's one less on your journey.**

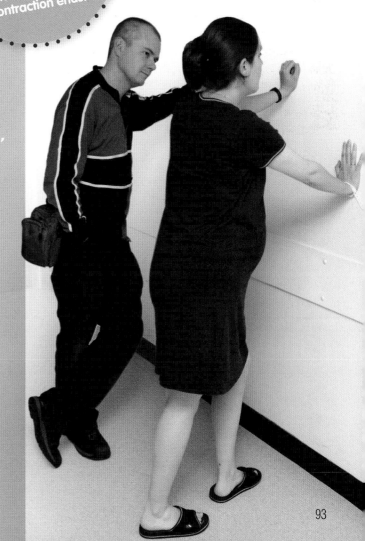

Checks and **monitoring** during labour

Wear something cool and comfortable like an old T-shirt.

Both you and your baby will be checked regularly throughout labour to make sure you're both OK.

Everything from your blood pressure and temperature to your urine and pulse will be assessed throughout the first stage.

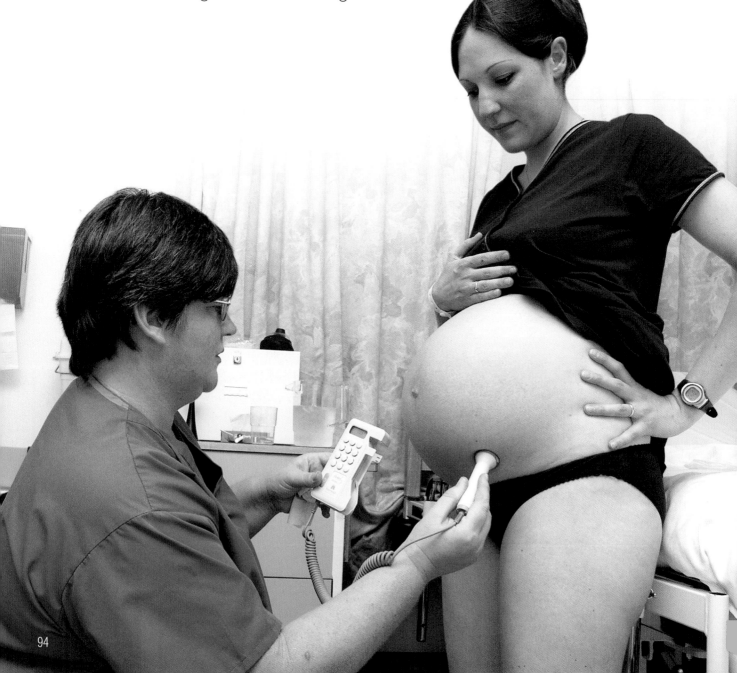

How your baby may be monitored

Measuring her heart rate is a way of assessing your baby's health and strength throughout labour and birth.

Different ways of monitoring

○ A Pinard stethoscope is a type of ear-trumpet placed against your abdomen to listen to your baby's heart. It is used from time to time during labour.

○ A Doppler is a small portable machine using ultrasound for monitoring at intervals. A small transmitter–receiver is placed on your abdomen to pick up the heartbeat.

○ Electronic fetal monitoring (EFM) uses ultrasound waves to transmit your baby's heart rate to a machine via a 'transducer' held against your abdomen. Alternatively, a small electrode can be clipped onto your baby's scalp (or bottom, in a breech baby) and this picks up and transmits the heartbeat. The heart rate usually appears in digital form on the screen, and a record is traced on graph paper and printed out.

○ Telemetry uses the same sort of transducer or scalp electrode, but sends signals by radio waves to the receiver. You're not actually attached to the monitor by wires, so you are free to move around as long as you stay within its range.

> Although it seemed to happen slowly, it was brilliant to be there from the beginning. I really felt involved.
> *Geoff, Perth*

Electronic fetal monitoring

EFM monitors the baby continuously. For some babies this can be important – if the baby is at risk or if it's known that there may be a problem.

In most cases, continuous EFM is not very useful in uncomplicated labour. Interpreting the monitor reading is a highly skilled job. Even very experienced obstetricians differ in opinion about what is a 'normal' reading, and what may give cause for concern. In many hospitals, midwives agree that continuous EFM is not needed for normal labour, especially in the first stage.

EFM is necessary when an intervention such as induction, or an epidural, is undertaken as these may cause stress to the baby. If you and your carers expect everything to be normal, you may prefer to have the other forms of monitoring with a Doppler or a Pinard stethoscope. You'll probably find your baby's heart is listened to every 15 or 20 minutes, and after most contractions in the second stage.

Checks you will have

You can expect the following things to be assessed regularly throughout the first stage:

• your blood pressure, pulse and temperature

• your urine (to help check your energy levels)

• the length, strength and frequency of your contractions

• possibly your cervix through an internal or vaginal examination.

Transition

An intense stage of the birth, sometimes referred to as 'transition', comes between the first and second stages. Many women clearly experience it as different from other parts of their labour. You may feel an urge to push or you may feel that your labour has stopped altogether.

Your midwife will guide you through this stage, helping you through your contractions and encouraging you to find the best position.

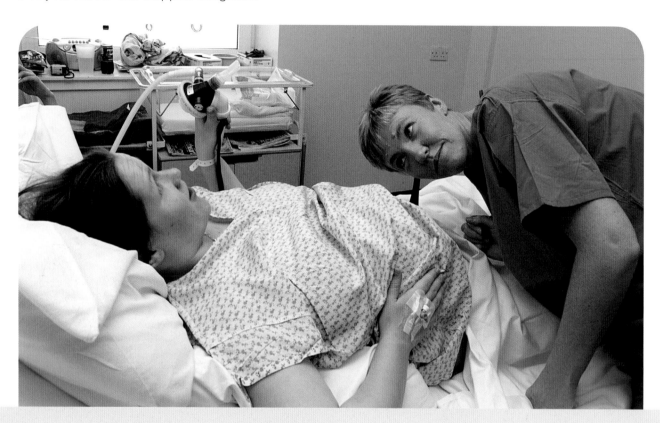

transition: what you can expect

Transition is a psychological state as well as a physical one and it can be very intense. You may feel impatient, tired, irritable and even angry and frustrated with your carers and birthing partner. This is a perfectly natural reaction and it means that the birth of your baby is not far off.

○ Remember it's OK to let everyone know how you are feeling.

○ If you don't want anyone to touch you, including your birthing partner, let them know.

○ Using the breathing techniques you have learned may help keep you calm between contractions.

○ Your partner should know not to take your frustrations and irritability too personally – you're both nearly there!

the **second stage**

This is the stage where your baby actually arrives. It starts when your cervix is fully dilated and ends with the birth of your baby. With a first baby, the second stage can last between ten minutes and two hours or even longer. It's easier with your second baby.

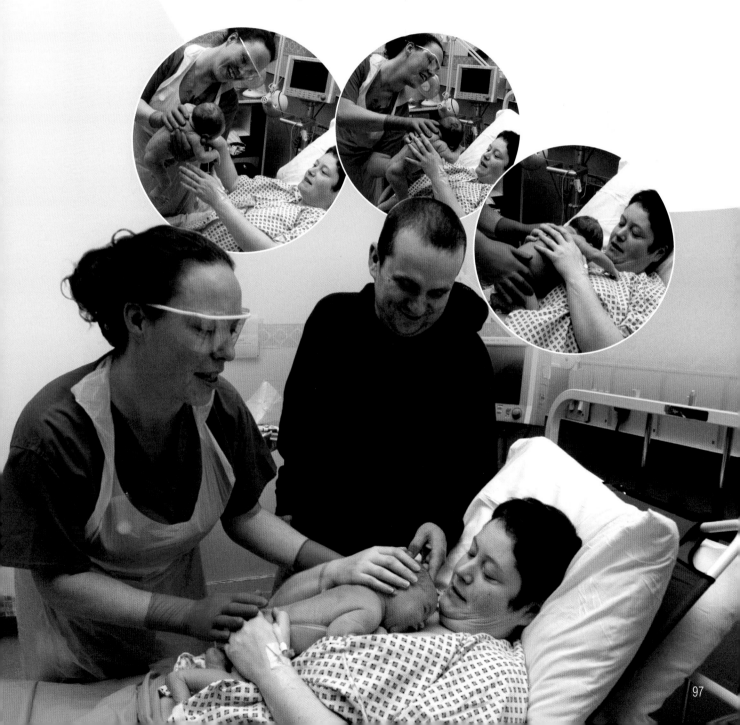

Giving birth to your baby

At this stage, contractions are helping to push your baby out. You may want to try different positions at this point and find the one that feels best for you.

What you can do

When you reach the second stage, you will probably feel a powerful urge to push. This is called bearing down.

You may want to push about three times in each contraction. You may feel when the time is right to push, or your midwife will guide you. If you have had an epidural for pain relief *(see page 73),* you may not feel the urge to bear down as strongly, so your midwife will tell you when you should push.

Some women like to hold their breath when they are pushing but it's important not to hold it for too long.

As your baby's head stretches the birth canal and the perineum (the area of skin between the vagina and the anus), you may feel a powerful burning sensation, which normally lasts only a few minutes.

Your midwife is crucial at this stage. She will guide you through the labour, encouraging you and helping you and your partner in the last minutes before the birth.

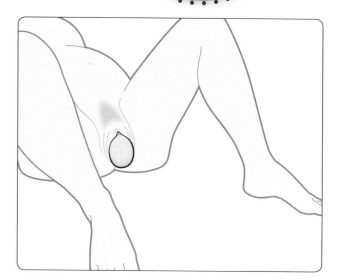

You will feel your perineum stretch at this point. If there's a risk of tearing, you may be asked to stop pushing *(see episiotomy, opposite).* Instead, you may be asked to pant or push more gently to 'breathe the baby out'.

episiotomy

Sometimes the perineum doesn't stretch easily over the baby's head. Your midwife may suggest that she cuts the perineum to help with the birth of the baby's head. This cut is known as an 'episiotomy'. Before the procedure is performed, a local anaesthetic may be injected into the muscle to reduce the discomfort or pain during the procedure. Episiotomy is only done when necessary and is not a routine procedure so it will be discussed with you. You will need stitches after the birth.

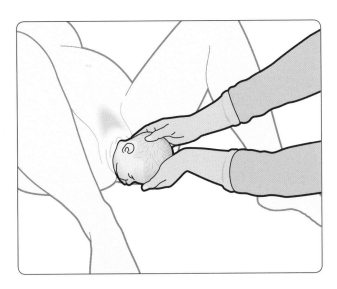

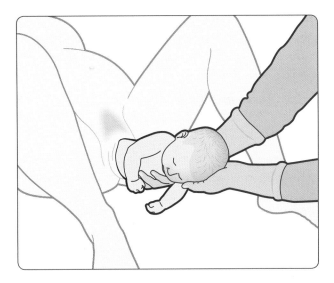

If a small tear in your perineum occurs it may need to be repaired after your baby is born. When her head can be seen completely at the vulva it is 'crowning'. This is a truly amazing moment. The midwife may encourage dad to have a first look at his new baby!

With the next couple of contractions, your baby's head comes out. The midwife may feel for the umbilical cord to make sure it's not around her neck. Your baby's shoulders will turn so that she's sideways on, facing your leg. The rest of her body then comes out quickly and easily. Your baby is born!

If you and your baby **need help**

Assisting birth

In some situations, an unplanned Caesarean section *(see pages 80–81)*, forceps or ventouse (vacuum) extraction are used to assist your baby's birth. These can happen for various reasons:

○ Your baby is short of oxygen – called fetal distress. This is diagnosed when the baby's heart rate slows in response to contractions, and doesn't speed up again as it should. A further sign is if the baby's bowels pass meconium (the contents of the bowels). This will stain the amniotic fluid a green or brown colour. A small blood sample may be taken from the baby's scalp to be measured for oxygen.

○ Your baby's exit is blocked or hampered – the position may be difficult, such as face-up (occipito-posterior), or your pelvis may not be able to open wide enough, sometimes due to your position.

○ Contractions have weakened.

○ Your baby is preterm, which means the head needs more protection.

○ You are too tired to push because of a long labour.

○ You have a condition such as a heart disorder, and should not push for too long.

If you need help with forceps or ventouse

Forceps and ventouse are both instruments that are attached to your baby's head so she can be pulled out. You will be given an anaesthetic, most likely an epidural or a spinal, or a local anaesthetic called a pudendal block. Your bladder may be emptied with a catheter which is a thin tube inserted into your bladder. You will probably need an episiotomy (*see page 99*) to allow room for the forceps to be inserted.

You will probably be helped to lie down on your back, and your legs will be raised in stirrups.

After the forceps have been inserted, as you feel each contraction coming, you push, just as you were doing before, as the doctor pulls. After the birth your baby may show bruising on each side of her head where the forceps have been.

Ventouse extraction can turn your baby for delivery. It uses a tube with a cup which attaches to the baby's head by suction. You push with each contraction and the doctor pulls.

Ventouse extraction can cause swelling (sometimes called a 'chignon') on your baby's head. This is not permanent, and will disappear over the next few days.

> ### How you may be feeling
> Sometimes women feel disappointed if they've had a Caesarean birth. You may feel you have missed out on something or be feeling guilty because you didn't manage to give birth without assistance. Understanding why you needed a Caesarean section can help you put the experience in perspective. Talk about your feelings with your midwife and other mothers who have had Caesarean births. The important thing is that you and your baby are safe and well.

First moments

Soon after the birth, your midwife will assess your baby's wellbeing – checking your baby's breathing, colour, muscle tone, response to stimulation and heart rate. This is called the Apgar score *(see page 105)*.

Your baby may look a little squashed and wrinkly at first and possibly blueish on her head and feet.

How your baby looks

○ She may have creamy vernix on her skin.

○ Her skin may be blotchy or have dry flaky patches.

○ There may be a few streaks of blood (yours, from your tear or episiotomy if you had one).

○ Her head may look a funny shape – the soft skull bones have moulded themselves to make it easier to squeeze through the birth canal. It'll look less misshapen soon.

○ She'll have blue eyes though this may not be their final colour.

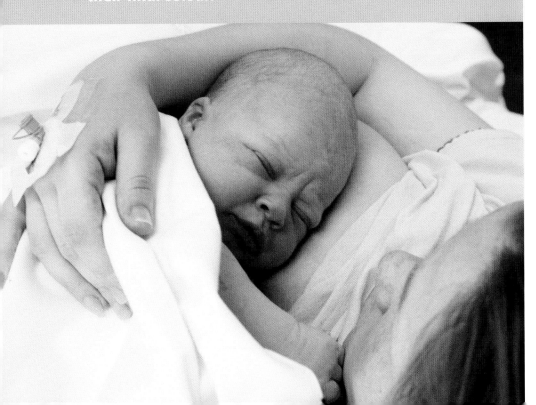

Skin-to-skin

You will be encouraged to hold your baby immediately after she is born, provided everything is OK with both of you. Cuddle her close without anything between you.

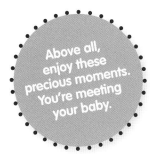

Above all, enjoy these precious moments. You're meeting your baby.

Getting to know each other

This close contact helps your baby stay warm; she'll be hearing your heartbeat as she did in the womb; her circulation will be better and she's less likely to cry. What's more, skin-to-skin contact has been shown to help get breastfeeding off to a good start.

Skin-to-skin with you is best until your baby has had a good first feed, but if you are unwell the next best thing is for your baby to have skin-to-skin contact with your partner.

> The first time I saw our son, he was tiny and squashed but so, so special.
> *Vijay, Glasgow*

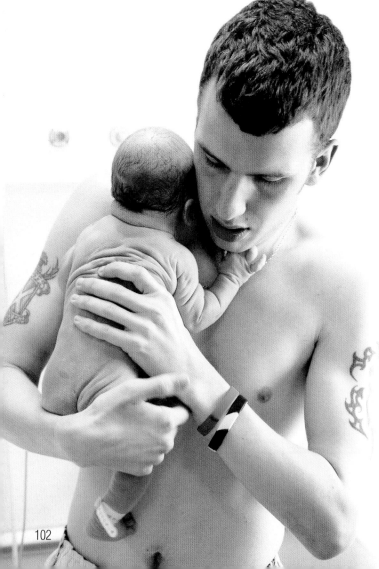

the **third stage**

The third stage of labour includes the delivery of the placenta and membranes after your baby has been born, and the control of bleeding.

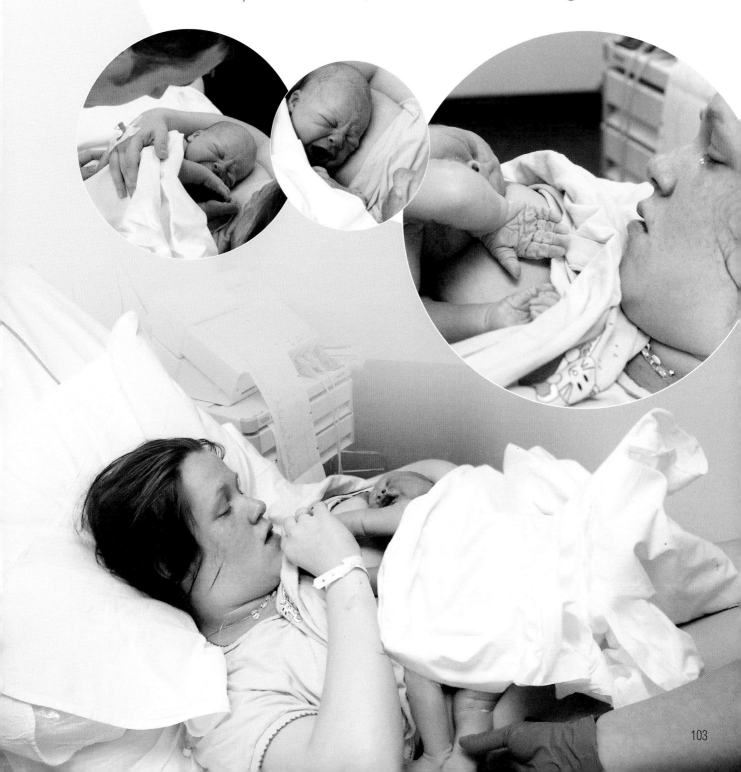

Routine actions in the third stage

For many women, you may not even be aware what is going on – you'll be too busy getting to know your baby.

In most hospital units, the third stage is 'actively managed', which may speed up this stage of labour. However, you may choose a physiological, 'unaided' third stage.

Physiological third stage

An unaided or physiological third stage happens without an injection or cord traction and can take longer than an 'actively managed' third stage. The action of breastfeeding your baby, or simply having her lie on your chest with skin-to-skin contact, stimulates the release of the hormone oxytocin. This helps your uterus to contract and push out the placenta and the membranes. The cord is cut when it stops pulsating, often after the placenta is delivered.

You may want to discuss the third stage and whether it is actively managed or not when making your birth plan. If you have problems in the first or second stages of your labour (or with a previous birth) then a physiological third stage may not be a safe option. Discuss this with your midwife.

Complications

- Occasionally, the placenta does not detach from the uterus. When this happens, the mother needs a small operation (under anaesthetic) to remove it.

- Sometimes women will bleed severely during the third stage. This is called postpartum haemorrhage or PPH and needs to be treated immediately.

Routine 'actively managed' third stage

- You may have an injection to cause the uterus to contract or shrink. This is given when the baby is being born, usually when the first shoulder is coming out. The injection will go into your thigh or buttock and the midwife will ask your permission first.

- Once your baby is born, the umbilical cord is clamped and cut.

- As the injection takes effect, it stimulates the uterus into contracting, causing the placenta to detach. At this stage, you may be able to push the placenta out. More usually, the midwife will help deliver it by putting a hand on your tummy to protect the uterus and keeping the cord taut (this is called 'cord traction').

- The placenta comes away and the blood vessels that were 'holding on' to it close off as the muscle in your uterus contracts. This prevents bleeding – although it's normal to bleed a little. You may feel the placenta slide down and out between your legs, followed by the membranes.

After the birth

You may hardly be aware of the third stage, as you will be focused on your baby. Seeing and handling your baby, and offering her your breast will stimulate hormones that help the placenta to separate. You may feel shaky due to adrenaline and the adjustments your body immediately starts to make, or you may simply be on a high. You may find it hard to pay attention to the baby if you have had a long labour. There's nothing wrong with your maternal instincts; you are simply exhausted. If this happens to you, take your time. After a rest you will be much more interested in getting to know your baby. A lot of women are very hungry and ready for tea and toast, while others want to telephone everyone and tell them the wonderful news!

Admire your new baby. Count her fingers and toes. Hold her close to your body, preferably skin-to-skin. If you're too tired, your partner can hold her against his chest. If you're going to breastfeed, offer your breast as soon as possible; your midwife will help you. Don't worry if your baby doesn't seem very interested. Even if she's only touching and nuzzling you, this will help her to get going with breastfeeding.

> **The support I had from everyone, especially the midwives, was fantastic. It's given me the confidence to think, "Yes, I can do this!"**
> *Joanne, Falkirk*

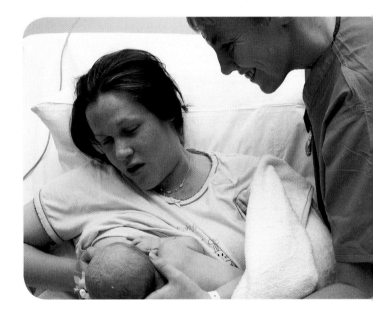

your baby's Apgar score

At birth your midwife assesses your baby's wellbeing with the Apgar score, by observation, usually at one minute and five minutes. Some units do a two-minute assessment only. Your baby's breathing, colour, muscle tone, response to stimulation and heart rate are checked, and given a mark of zero, one, or two for these aspects of your baby's appearance and health.

Some blood may be taken from the blood vessels in your baby's umbilical cord after birth. This is to check the level of oxygen in your baby's blood at the time of birth. You should ask your midwife if you have any questions about this.

Being in **hospital;** going **back home**

The first 24 hours

Some mums enjoy their time in hospital while others find it stressful and can't wait to get home. By the time you go home, however, you will have been shown the basics of baby care, including bathing, feeding and keeping your baby safe.

Most maternity units now recommend that babies stay with their mums 24 hours a day in hospital, called 'rooming in'. This helps with feeding and bonding. It also reduces the risk of infection.

Giving birth can be an exhausting experience, so you may not want visits from anyone but those closest to you. Don't be afraid to say you're not up to lots of visitors – partners and grandparents can be helpful in suggesting people don't come to visit until later.

Within the first 10 days

You'll usually be visited several times at home during the first 10 days. Some new parents need to be seen more than others and additional support will be provided for babies who have special needs or who needed treatment in the neonatal intensive care unit.

Your midwife will record your baby's weight during the first 10 days of her life and also carry out a newborn blood spot test *(see page 116)*. She will record the feeding method you have chosen for your baby and answer any questions you may have.

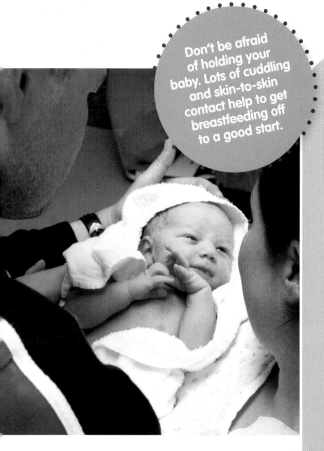

Don't be afraid of holding your baby. Lots of cuddling and skin-to-skin contact help to get breastfeeding off to a good start.

Screening in the first 72 hours or first three days of life

When your baby is born the midwife will begin a series of screening tests which will include checking the:

- palate
- hips for signs of dislocation
- eyes
- cardiovascular system
- genitalia
- femoral pulses.

Your baby's birthweight, head circumference and length will also be recorded.

Professional questionnaire

You can help your hospital by answering a questionnaire that a health professional may give you. The information you provide will help them continually improve the care that they give to mums in labour.

You can choose whether or not you take part and all the information will be kept strictly confidential.

> I was just overwhelmed with joy – we both were. I fell head-over-heels in love with Jamie as soon as I saw him. He seemed to stare at us, and we were both talking to him, stroking and touching him… then after this he fell asleep so peacefully, for about two hours. I was on a high for at least two days.
>
> *Katie, Edinburgh*

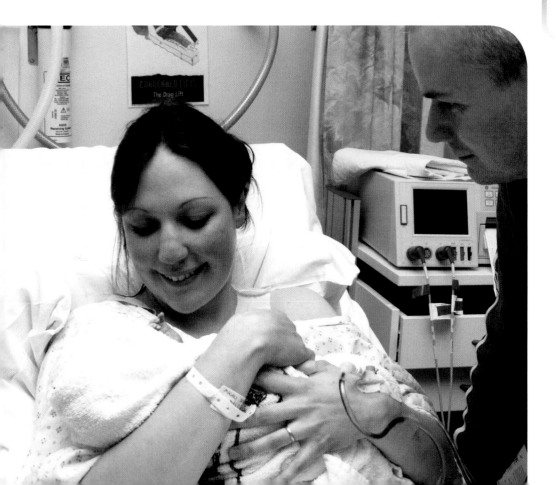

at a glance

✳ Your midwife will check both you and your baby after the birth.

✳ Your baby's wellbeing is immediately measured by the midwife by checking her heart rate, breathing, muscle tone, skin colour and response to stimulus.

✳ You can begin bonding with her right away.

you and your baby's first days together

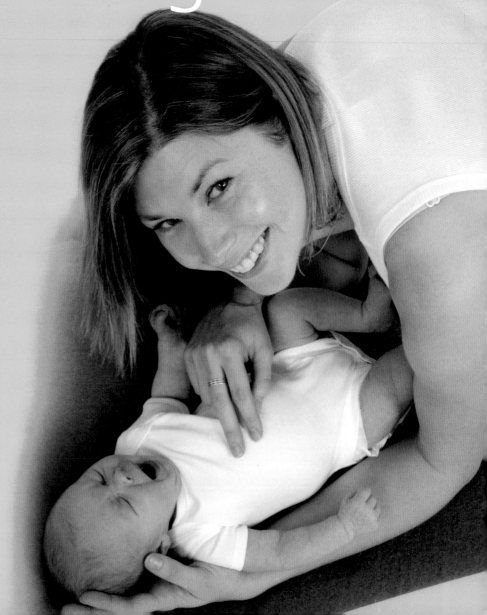

Section 3

Getting to know your baby

It's what you've spent the last nine months waiting for – meeting and getting to know your baby!

Some babies sleep a lot, others are wakeful. Some want to feed all the time, others don't. It's all normal. Contact your midwife, health visitor/public health nurse if you have concerns.

How you may feel

New parents can react in different ways. Some may fall 'head-over-heels in love' with their baby straight away. Others will take a bit longer. You will probably be both excited and exhausted and it may take a while to get used to your new baby and to figure out everything she wants and needs.

Partners may feel a bit left out at this point, especially if they are leaving mum and baby in hospital to go home. But it's important to involve your partner in supporting you, as well as getting to know the newest member of the family.

How your baby looks

At first she may look a bit odd! She may look squashed, wrinkly and even bruised from the birth. She may have 'stork marks' – red markings which disappear within a few days. Possibly her hands and feet will look blueish. This is all perfectly normal. Within the next few days, her skin will smooth out a little, her head will become rounder and the vernix (the creamy white substance that protected her skin in the womb) will disappear.

Bonding with your baby

What does bonding mean? Well, child experts describe bonding as the very intense feelings of attachment you develop for your baby. You may feel an almost overwhelming sense of love and affection – and a strong desire to care for and protect her. For some mums (and dads!) this can happen straight away. For others it can take days, or even weeks.

Bonding is a very individual experience and you shouldn't worry if it doesn't happen immediately. Remember that your baby is a completely new little person, and however cute she is, it takes time to get to know her. True parent-child bonding develops and strengthens through caring for your baby every day. You'll find that your feelings deepen over time.

Skin-to-skin contact

Touch is incredibly important for babies. That's why your baby is placed on your tummy as soon as possible after she is born. This skin-to-skin contact not only helps you and your baby to bond, but can comfort her when she is upset. Remember that your baby loves to be touched and that it's a critical part of her emotional growth and development.

For both parents, the main thing is to get used to looking after your new baby – being close to her, talking to her, holding and cuddling her. This increases your confidence as a parent and also gives your baby the best emotional start in life.

This early relationship lays a very important foundation for your baby's wellbeing and development. Babies who have a secure bond with their mother usually go on to be confident children who are less prone to mental health problems.

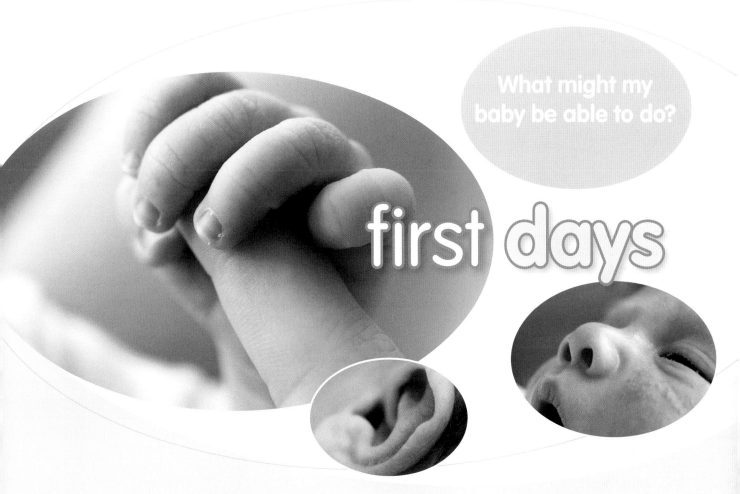

What might my baby be able to do?

first days

Your baby can see in black, white and grey from the moment she is born, although she finds it difficult to focus on anything more than about 25 cm away. It does mean that she can see your face when you hold her in your arms and she may even hold your gaze for a few moments.

She can also hear and be startled by loud noises. Babies seem to like soft voices best, the kind of tone most of us would use anyway when talking to a new baby.

Your baby will recognise your voice, and speaking to her will help develop a two-way relationship, which is important for her future social skills.

She can grasp. Try touching the palm of her hand or stroking her feet. Play and communicate with your baby as much as you can; talk to her, smile at her, laugh with her and watch her reactions develop.

Your baby can smell – she'll recognise the smell of your body and that makes her feel secure. After your baby is born, have skin-to-skin contact first, and feed your baby, before you have a shower.

Most of all, she'll love being cuddled close to you because she's been used to being in a confined space in the womb, and this makes her feel safe. You'll enjoy it too!

Changes in your body

Giving birth can be an exhausting experience which brings about all sorts of physical and emotional changes. The first few days may be tough – so don't be too hard on yourself.

The first few days

For the first few days after the birth, you may feel really tired. If you had a Caesarean section you'll be recovering from the operation. If you've had stitches, the affected areas may be sore and you might be worried about going to the toilet. Although you may have expected to feel great, you might actually feel a bit down *(see opposite)*.

Immediately after the birth, your tummy will look saggy and soft. As your uterus shrinks back to its pre-pregnancy size in the few days after the birth, you may feel contractions known as 'afterpains', especially if you're breastfeeding. If you find these uncomfortable ask your midwife, GP or pharmacist what pain relief is safe to take, if you need it.

Your breasts may swell and feel tender when your milk comes in *(see page 122)*. A well-fitted bra should help support your breasts and again you can take pain relief (recommended by your midwife, GP or pharmacist) if necessary.

You might be constipated for the first couple of days after giving birth – not helped by worrying about stitches! The best thing you can do to make it easier is drink lots of water and eat high-fibre foods including fruit and vegetables *(see page 124)*. It's unlikely you'll damage your stitches but you can hold a pad over your perineum when you try to go – and avoid straining!

If your stitches are very sore, speak to your midwife who can recommend safe pain relief. You can also make the stitched area feel better by bathing in warm water and drying carefully.

Lochia and bleeding

For the next three to four weeks, sometimes longer, you'll have a discharge from your vagina, called 'lochia'. Initially this is a bit like having a heavy period. At first it's bright red, then pinkish brown, then cream. The lochia will be heavy at first and you'll need lots of changes of sanitary towels (tampons aren't suitable because of the risk of infection). The discharge should slow down after the first week.

Get medical advice if you experience any of the following:

- you start to lose fresh red blood or your discharge seems too heavy

- the discharge gets smelly

- you have stomach pains or a temperature

- you pass clots after the first few days.

Remember, some fresh red blood loss is normal after a breastfeed but only in the first few days. If the discharge hasn't stopped after six weeks or so, speak to your health visitor/public health nurse or GP.

How you may be feeling

It's perfectly normal to feel a bit down after the birth. Around 70% of all new mums suffer from so-called 'baby blues'. Baby blues describes feelings of mild depression and tearfulness. This is quite different to post-natal depression (PND). It normally kicks in two to three days after the birth and shouldn't last very long. But it can happen at any time and may last for only a couple of hours or even up to a few days.

Baby blues and how it might affect you

Caring for a new baby can be exhausting. Poor sleep and worries about coping may upset your mood. You may feel really tired or generally not very well. You may cry for no particular reason and find it's impossible to cheer up. Little things that you'd normally take in your stride suddenly seem like huge problems.

We don't exactly know what causes the baby blues but we do know it's perfectly normal. There could be hormonal reasons. While you're pregnant, your body produces lots of hormones to help your baby develop. After the birth, levels of these hormones drop while others, needed to produce milk, rise. This hormonal rollercoaster can easily lead to mood changes.

The baby blues will go away but it's important to get extra support while it lasts and if these feelings don't pass within a few days, do talk to your midwife or health visitor/public health nurse.

at a glance

❋ Your body may take some time to recover from the birth.

❋ You breasts are larger as your milk comes in. They may be uncomfortable but should feel better soon.

❋ Breastfeeding helps your uterus shrink back to its pre-pregnancy size.

❋ You might be feeling tired, emotional and that you're not coping – this is very common.

❋ Around 70% of all new mums will suffer from 'baby blues' which can last up to a few days.

❋ If it lasts longer than 10 days or is particularly severe, seek help from your health visitor/public health nurse, or GP.

helping new mums

New mums need someone to listen to them, help with the baby and provide support and reassurance.

There's lots you can do to help:

- be ready to listen – and pass the tissues

- remind her that the baby blues are common and will pass

- make sure she isn't overwhelmed by visitors

- help with the baby

- offer to do the cleaning, cooking and ironing

- try and ensure she gets as much rest as possible.

Tests you will be offered for your baby

In the first days after the birth, you will be offered various tests to make sure your baby is healthy. The doctor or midwife will discuss the tests with you beforehand and will be happy to answer any questions. Although these tests are recommended, it's up to you whether you decide to have them done.

Routine examinations

You will be offered two physical examinations of your baby after she is born. The first is carried out immediately after the birth. The second is called the routine examination of the newborn and usually takes place 24 hours after your baby is born – although it can be any time between six and 72 hours after birth.

This examination will be carried out by a children's doctor (paediatrician), specially trained midwife or a neonatal nurse. They will examine your baby from top to toe, and in particular will examine her head, heart, hips, eyes and genitalia.

It is important that you inform the person carrying out the examination of any problems that run in the family – both on your side, and the baby's father's side – such as dislocated hips as a child, heart conditions, sight or hearing defects. They also need to know about any difficulties you experienced during pregnancy or at your antenatal scans – or if your baby was lying breech. If a problem is found, your baby might need further tests, or to be seen again at an outpatients' clinic after she has been discharged from hospital.

Heart check

If you are told your baby's heart makes an additional sound, called a 'murmur', you may feel worried, but in fact the condition is very common. One estimate is that 50% of babies have a heart murmur in the first week. Within a few weeks, most murmurs are not heard any more.

Developmental dysplasia of hips

The midwife or doctor will examine each hip joint to check that the head of the thigh bone (femur) moves as it should do within the socket at the hip, and that it doesn't slip out.

Undescended testes

For baby boys, the midwife will examine the scrotum to ensure that the testes (testicles) have travelled down from the abdomen. The testes usually move down into the scrotum two months before birth, but in some baby boys this does not happen. The 'undescended' testes may still descend in the first six months or up to one year after birth. If there is any concern about the testes at your baby's six to eight week check your health professional will arrange for your baby to be reviewed again. If you have any concerns about your baby's testes, for example a swelling, please seek medical advice.

Tests, checks and screening

A few routine checks for minor health problems will be carried out in the days and weeks after your baby is born. These are designed to set your mind at rest and to give your baby a good start in life.

Jaundice

The usual check is just to observe the skin, which is yellowish if the baby is jaundiced – many new babies have mild jaundice. If the yellow colour of the skin doesn't go away in a few days a blood check is done to see whether the jaundice is severe. Babies who are still jaundiced at 14 days will always be referred to a paediatrician for further investigations. There are other less common causes of jaundice which need to be ruled out. Most babies, however, are perfectly well.

Group B Streptococcus (Strep B)

This is a germ carried by up to one-third of mothers, and it usually doesn't cause any harm. However, it can be passed to the baby during labour, and a few babies who catch it will become very sick if they are not treated. Babies who are infected will be given antibiotics to prevent them from becoming ill. In some areas, routine testing for Strep B in mothers is being considered. Ask your midwife about local policy.

Newborn hearing screening

A simple screening test will be done within the first few weeks after your baby is born, maybe even before you leave the maternity unit, to check if your baby has a hearing loss. This is important for your baby's development and it means that you can get support and information at an early stage. If your baby's hearing is not tested, ask your midwife, health visitor/public health nurse, to make an appointment.

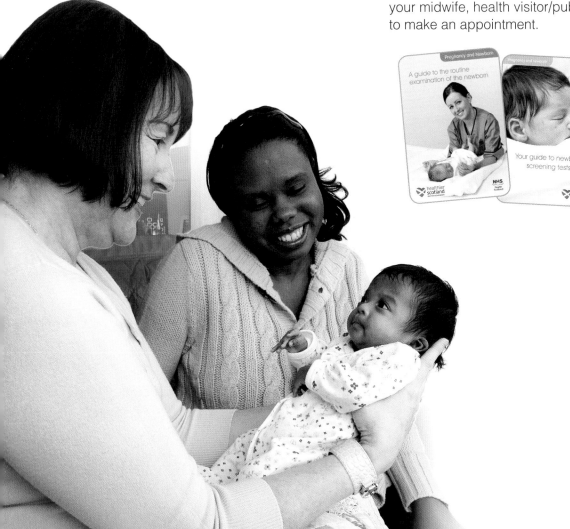

The newborn blood spot test

Although most babies are born healthy, a few may have problems. All babies are examined carefully after birth so that these can be picked up as early as possible. Some problems which can't be picked up in this way, will show up in the blood spot screening test. The blood spot test or 'heel prick test' is usually carried out when your baby is five days old. The midwife takes several spots of blood from the baby's heel and places them on a special card which is sent to the lab for testing for three rare conditions: Phenylketonuria (PKU), Congenital Hypothyroidism (CHT) and Cystic Fibrosis (CF).

Your midwife will explain the test and ask for consent to carry it out. If you choose not to let your baby have the test, you will be asked to sign a form confirming that the reasons for testing have been explained to you, and that you understand that a delay in diagnosis of these conditions may lead to permanent damage to your baby.

Normal results are not routinely reported to each family but your midwife or health visitor/public health nurse will be able to give you this information. If the test shows up an abnormal result, a hospital appointment will be arranged and your GP will be contacted.

Phenylketonuria (PKU)

This disorder affects around one in every 8,000 babies born in Scotland. Babies with this condition cannot process a substance called phenylalanine, which is present in many foods that contain protein, such as milk, meat, fish, cheese and cereals.

If PKU is detected by the test, your baby will be seen by a paediatrician as soon as possible and further tests will be carried out before a final diagnosis is made. If PKU is diagnosed, your baby must be given a special diet which will help her to develop normally.

If a baby with PKU is not screened, the condition will remain undetected. Babies who have PKU and who are not treated, will gradually develop irreversible brain damage.

Congenital Hypothyroidism (CHT)

This condition affects around one in every 3,500 babies born in Scotland. It means that a baby is born unable to produce enough of the hormone thyroxine. This hormone is vital for normal mental and physical development. It is easily treated by giving thyroxine by mouth but, if it is not detected and treated, a lack of thyroxine can lead to slower than normal growth and severe learning difficulties.

Cystic Fibrosis (CF)

This is a serious inherited condition which affects one in every 2,500 babies born in Scotland. It can affect the pancreas and the lungs. Poor digestion and absorption of foods and chest infections are common problems. The majority of affected babies will be picked up by the blood spot test but it is necessary to carry out further tests before a final diagnosis can be made.

Early treatment for Cystic Fibrosis may help prevent the long-term complications of this disease. It will also help affected children by maintaining good nutrition, minimising chest infections and improving quality of life.

Ask your midwife for more information and a copy of the leaflet *A parent's guide to newborn blood spot screening.*

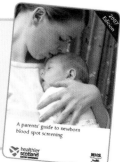

Babies who need extra care

Some babies (around one in eight) are admitted to specialist neonatal units or children's hospitals because they arrive earlier than expected or are too sick to cope on their own. If this happens to your baby, you may not be able to take her home with you.

Staying in hospital

Your baby might need the special care of the neonatal (newborn) unit or children's hospital. These wards have special equipment as well as specially trained staff to care for the babies on them. The length of a baby's stay can vary from days to months and depends on each baby's needs. Most children's hospitals and neonatal units can make arrangements for parents to either stay with their baby or to be close by.

Coming home

Once a baby who needs extra care has come home, you will probably stay in touch with the hospital paediatrician either directly or through a community neonatal nurse who specialises in newborn babies.

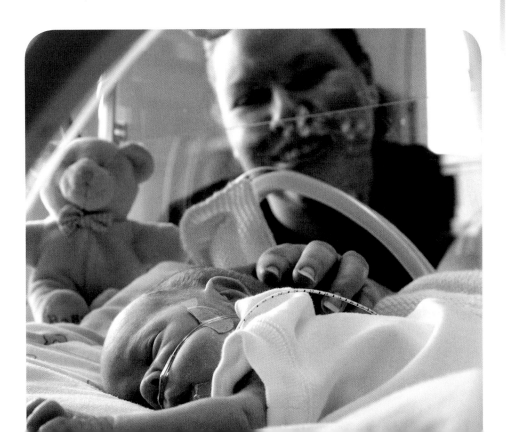

at a glance

* Your baby will be offered routine examinations to make sure she's OK.

* You have the right to choose whether you want your baby to have these tests or not.

* Tests, checks and screening are designed to set your mind at rest.

* Some babies may need extra care – for example if they are born very early.

Going **home**

You'll probably have mixed feelings about going home. It's normal to be both excited and nervous. Remember you will have support from your midwife and your health visitor/public health nurse at home.

How long you'll stay in hospital

Hospitals in different parts of the country have different policies. However, if mum and baby are both doing well, you'll usually be getting ready to go home somewhere between six and 24 hours after giving birth, depending on how you are feeling. If you've had a Caesarean section or if you or your baby need extra care, you might need to stay in hospital for a bit longer.

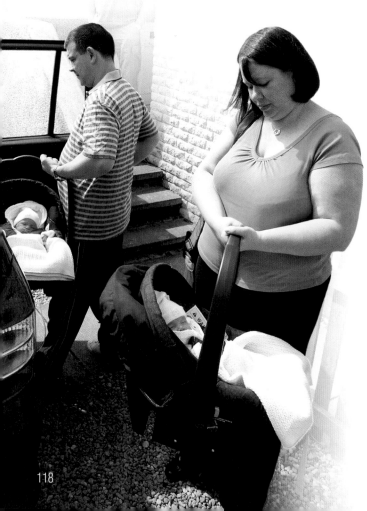

Confidentiality and your notes

In Scotland, mums look after their own medical notes. You'll take these notes home from hospital with you and they'll be used by your midwife and then your health visitor/public health nurse to ensure that you and your baby get the best possible support.

Although your notes are completely confidential, if there is any aspect of your health – or your baby's – which would benefit from the input of another specialist, your GP, midwife or health visitor/public health nurse is allowed to share that information.

Getting support

You may want to arrange some support for the first few days at home. It may sound obvious, but partners, friends or family can help by making sure there's a clean and tidy house to come home to, rather than a sink full of dishes and a washing machine waiting to be emptied. Also that there's food in the fridge and the toilet is clean! You will want your home to be a safe and welcoming place for the newest member of the family. That includes making sure there's a safe place to change your baby, where she can't fall.

Support from healthcare professionals after the birth

In the first 10 days after you've given birth, you'll be looked after by a midwife both in hospital and at home. After this you'll be transferred into the care of a health visitor or public health nurse. You'll also need to register your baby with a GP.

The role of the health visitor

Your health visitor or public health nurse takes over your care from the midwife 10 days after the birth of your baby. He or she can be a real source of support and information and has a great deal of experience in looking after families with babies and children. He or she will invite you and your baby to attend a child health clinic where you can ask questions, discuss baby care and have your baby's health and growth checked. You may also be given a Personal Child Health Record (the Red Book) for you to write down information about your baby's growth, development, tests and immunisations. You should take this with you to any appointments with healthcare professionals. Your health visitor/public health nurse will be on hand and will support you as your confidence as a new parent grows – he or she may give you a number to call if you ever need any advice about your baby.

at a glance

❋ You'll probably get home within 24 hours of the birth but this varies.

❋ Midwives will show you how to care for your baby before you go home or once you are home.

❋ It's normal to feel nervous the first few nights at home but it does get better!

❋ Remember, you can ask your healthcare professional for advice and support.

❋ You will be given a Red Book as a main record of your child's health, growth and development.

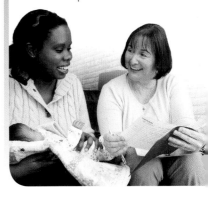

the child health programme

The Child Health Programme is the series of health checks, visits and immunisations that are offered to every child in Scotland from birth. They are carried out by healthcare professionals – usually GPs, midwives, health visitors, public health nurses and school nurses. Other specialists may be involved in hearing and sight checks.

The Child Health Programme is there to help you give your child the best start in life. It includes immunisations and routine checks for any health problems that your child may have, so that care or treatment can be arranged as soon as possible.

It also provides important opportunities for you to talk to a healthcare professional about your child's and family's health.

Feeding your baby

Whether you choose to breast or formula feed your baby, there is support and advice to help you get started. This section gives you lots of information to help you make an informed choice. It's really important that you are prepared, and feel confident about how to feed your baby.

Bonding through feeding

Feeding can be a very special time for mum and baby. It gives you the opportunity to hold your baby close and really get to know her. You might enjoy stroking her cheek or hands as she feeds and find that this is one of the best ways to enjoy precious time together and to develop a really strong emotional bond. Always hold your baby when you are feeding and enjoy this quiet, gentle time together.

You might find that feeding your baby gives you greater confidence as a new mum – particularly as you start to see her gain weight and fill out – that's all down to you! And as you both get the hang of feeding, it will be a time that you'll both look forward to.

Your baby's appetite

In the early days, your baby's tummy is very small – only about the size of a ping pong ball. So, at this stage, she may want to feed every couple of hours. You'll also find that some days she may want more milk than others. That's all perfectly normal.

Feeding cues

When your baby is hungry, you will see her 'root' – that is, she'll turn her head and open her mouth, looking for food. She may also bring her hands up to her mouth, and stick out her tongue or make sucking faces. This is your cue to settle down for a feed!

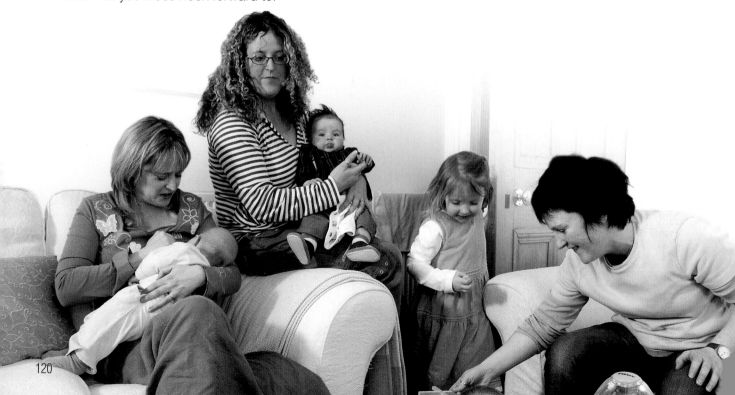

Feeding patterns

Early on, your baby with feed little and often – she will feed, sleep and have wakeful periods according to her own little body clock – and the best way to deal with this is to go with the flow. For example, if you're tired, snatch a quick sleep when she does.

Are you sitting comfortably?

Whether you breastfeed or bottle feed, it's important to get yourself comfortable for this special time. After all, you could be feeding for a while. Try out some different options. You may have a favourite chair or sofa, or find that sitting up in bed with lots of pillows behind your back works best for you. Do make sure that your back is well supported and that you hold your baby close.

Atmosphere is also important – especially in the early days. Choose somewhere that you feel calm, relaxed and comfortable – and where you have easy access to the television, telephone and a cold drink or snack.

Your right to feed

An Act was passed by the Scottish Parliament in 2005 which makes it an offence to prevent anyone feeding a baby in a public place. So, once you're ready to go out and about with your baby, do remember that you have the right to feed her milk in public at any time – this includes anywhere the public have general access such as cafes, buses, parks or GP surgeries. And this is true whether you are bottle feeding or breastfeeding.

If you would like to eat peanuts or foods containing peanuts (such as peanut butter) while breastfeeding, you can choose to do so as part of a healthy balanced diet, unless you are allergic to them or your health professional has advised you not to. If you have a child under six months and are not breastfeeding (you are feeding your baby formula milk), then there is no reason why you should avoid eating peanuts or foods containing peanuts.

How to tell if your baby is feeding well

Healthy, well-nourished babies have five to six wet nappies every day and pass soft, yellow stools after the first few days, if they are breastfed. The odd green stool is not significant in a breastfed baby. For both breast and bottle fed babies, nappies are a great indicator of health!

Babies should be able to pass stools easily and regularly. Well-nourished babies seem alert and healthy, and are comfortable and satisfied after feeding.

Some babies don't gain weight as fast as others. Occasionally this can be because they aren't getting enough milk but usually it is simply because each baby is different.

Is my baby getting enough milk?

If you are at all worried about your baby's appetite or feeding, do speak to your midwife, health visitor/public health nurse. Here are some things to check for:

- Is your baby feeding at least six to eight times a day (for the first two to three weeks)?
- Can you see her swallowing while she feeds?
- If you are breastfeeding do your breasts soften after feeds?
- If your baby was jaundiced, has her yellow colour gone?
- Is your baby back up to her birthweight?
- Does your baby have at least six to eight heavy wet nappies over 24 hours (after the 5th day) and is her pee pale and odourless?
- Is your baby having dirty nappies at least once a day that are (after the 5th day) yellowy-mustard in colour?

Breastfeeding

Your breast milk provides all the goodness and nutrients your baby needs and will give her the best start in life. Not only does breast milk carry your antibodies – which will help to give her immunity against common illnesses like colds and coughs – but breastfeeding is good for you too. And remember, only a mother can make breast milk!

Establishing breastfeeding can take a while, but the benefits will last you a lifetime!

Good for baby, good for you

Medical research suggests that the longer you breastfeed, the more benefits it brings you. These include a lower risk of ovarian cancer, breast cancer and hip fractures in later life. Breastfeeding may also help you return to your pre-pregnancy weight and babies who are breastfed are less likely to be obese in later life or to develop eczema, asthma or childhood diabetes.

It is now recommended that babies are exclusively breastfed for the first six months, in other words, it is not necessary to give your baby any other food or drink.

Practice makes perfect

Although breastfeeding is a completely natural process, it's still one that both mum and baby have to learn. Breastfeeding gets easier – for you and your baby – with practise. Keep this in mind and stick at it. Both in hospital and at home, ask for support from your midwife and health visitor/public health nurse. They'll be able to offer practical help to ensure that your baby is properly attached to your breast *(see pages 126–127)* and feeding well, as well as giving you lots of tips to help you both get the best out of breastfeeding.

In the early days while you're establishing breastfeeding it's best not to give any bottles – even of expressed breast milk. This is because breast and bottle fed babies suck differently and introducing a bottle may be confusing.

When your milk comes in

Your breasts begin to produce a substance called colostrum while you are still pregnant and in the early days of breastfeeding. This is low in fat and high in carbohydrates, protein and antibodies to keep your baby healthy. Yellow to orange in colour, and thick and sticky in texture, it's extremely easy for your baby to digest, and therefore the perfect first food. Even a short period of breastfeeding will bring your baby benefits.

If you breastfeed your baby early on and often, your breasts will then begin to produce mature milk around the third or fourth day after you've given birth. Your milk will increase in volume and will generally begin to appear thinner and whiter (more opaque).

Baby-led or demand feeding

At the beginning of a breastfeed, your baby's thirst will be quenched. Let her feed for as long as she wants to satisfy her, and so that she gets all the nutrients she needs to grow well. Feeding this way also means that you will avoid blocked ducts and engorgement *(see page 124)*.

Once your baby comes off your first breast, or is no longer swallowing milk, offer your second breast. She may not always take it, but whether she does or not, always start her next feed with your second breast.

Q *I chose to formula feed my first baby, but now I'm pregnant again, I'd like to give breastfeeding a go. Can you give me some advice?*

A. First of all – congratulations on your decision. Breastfeeding will give your baby the best possible start in life – and it's good for you too! When your baby is born, your midwife – both in hospital and at home – will give you all the practical help and support you need to get started. This will make you feel more confident – and there's additional support available from breastfeeding councillors too. Visit **www.breastfeeding.nhs.uk** for more information and **www.breastfeedingcommunity.co.uk** to find out about support organisations. Good luck!

Breastfeeding is free and convenient.

Is my baby getting enough milk?

Especially in the early days of breastfeeding, you'll find it quite difficult to tell if your baby has had enough milk. You may find that you think you've finished feeding, and are just getting ready to settle her, when she wakes up again, ready for another go!

You can be reassured that your baby is likely to be getting enough milk if she:

- attaches well and is being fed on demand
- changes rhythm while sucking, pauses during the feed and starts again without prompting
- comes off the breast of her own accord, looking full, satisfied and sleepy
- and also if feeding is comfortable and painless for you.

You might find it helpful to let your baby feed from one breast first until she comes off looking sleepy and contented. At this point you can sit her up, or place her over your shoulder and gently rub her back to see if she burps. If she's still looking alert and hungry, offer her more milk. If she's not, then don't!

at a glance

❋ Breast milk provides perfect nutrition, changing according to your baby's needs and its quality remains high, even if you are unwell.

❋ Antibodies in breast milk help babies fight common infections and help boost their developing immune system.

❋ Your breast milk supplies everything your baby needs for food and drink for around six months.

❋ Breastfeeding may help you return to your pre-pregnancy weight.

❋ Mothers who breastfeed have a lower risk of ovarian cancer, breast cancer and hip fractures later in life.

Call the National Breastfeeding Helpline on 0300 100 0212. Lines are open 9.30 am to 9.30 pm every day of the year.

Calls to 0300 numbers cost no more than calls to UK numbers starting 01 and 02, and will be part of any inclusive minutes that apply to your provider and call package.

Breast care

When you're new to breastfeeding, you may find it a little strange and uncomfortable at first – until both you and your baby have got the hang of good attachment. However, if you find that your nipples or breasts are painful – or that breastfeeding is sore – do contact your midwife, health visitor/public health nurse or breastfeeding consultant for advice.

Nursing bras and breast pads

Wearing a good nursing bra will not only give your breasts the support they need, but also make it easier for you to breastfeed, as they usually open either fully or partially at the front. And because you might find that you leak a little milk between feeds, breast pads inserted inside your bra will help to soak this up – you can buy both washable and disposable kinds.

Engorged breasts and mastitis

Both mastitis and engorgement can happen to breastfeeding mums, often in the first few weeks of breastfeeding. Baby-led feeding and making sure your baby is properly attached will help with both. If you have signs of either speak to your midwife or health visitor/public health nurse straight away.

Engorgement

Your breasts can become engorged at any stage but it is most likely to happen if you miss feeds or your baby is not attached correctly. Your breasts will feel hot, heavy and painful and may be shiny and red. You may have a temperature and your baby will have difficulty attaching. Expressing milk will help by softening the breast.

Mastitis

This is most common two weeks after your baby is born when a small clot of milk can block one or more of your breast ducts causing your breast to feel painful and swollen.

You may also feel flu-like symptoms, and your breast may be tender and have a red, wedge shaped area. It's important that you do not stop breastfeeding if you have mastitis symptoms as this may make it worse. If you don't improve within six to eight hours you may need an antibiotic from your GP.

Eating for mum!

You can now eat all of the things that you weren't able to eat when you were pregnant *(see pages 20–21)*. However, avoid large amounts of caffeine as this may make your baby irritable.

Try to eat a healthy and varied diet, including plenty of fruit and vegetables, starchy foods such as bread and pasta, and plenty of fibre, protein and dairy foods. Also, remember to drink lots of water as breastfeeding can make you feel thirsty – and if you don't drink enough fluids, you may get constipated.

Alcohol and breastfeeding

When you drink, small amounts of alcohol pass into your breast milk. For this reason, it is important to limit the amount of alcohol you drink to no more than one to two units once or twice a week. Drinking more than this can affect the baby's development and cause feeding, sleeping and digesting problems. Alcohol can also affect your milk supply. If it's a special occasion and you know you are going to have a drink, consider expressing your milk in advance. To be on the safe side, you may want to avoid alcohol altogether while you are breastfeeding.

Expressing your own milk

Expressing milk from your breasts is a useful skill to learn and your midwife will show you how to do this, using either your hand or a special breast pump.

Why express milk?

There are a number of reasons for expressing milk:

- you may be unable to breastfeed, however much you want to – giving your baby your own breast milk, from a bottle, cup or spoon ensures she is getting all the natural nutrients she needs

- you may need to relieve engorgement by releasing a little milk from your breasts

- you may want to go out with your friends or family and leave your own breast milk for your babysitter to feed your baby.

Storing expressed milk

You should store your expressed breast milk in the fridge, in sterilised containers, for up to five days. However, if you wish to store it for longer then freeze your breast milk in ice cube trays or freezer bags. It's best to freeze in small quantities as it's less wasteful if your baby only needs a small amount. And it helps to label and date your milk so you can keep track of how long you've stored it for.

Your expressed breast milk (EBM) can be stored in the fridge for up to five days, the freezer compartment of the fridge for up to two weeks or the freezer for up to six months. Do make sure that your fridge and freezer are clean and maintain a reliable temperature of 4°C or lower for the fridge; -18°C or lower for the freezer.

Warming expressed milk

If you are using breast milk that you've previously expressed and stored in the fridge, follow these simple instructions for bringing it up to the right temperature for your baby:

- remove stored milk from the fridge just before it is needed

- re-warm by placing in a container of warm water

- shake the bottle to ensure the feed has heated evenly

- check the feeding temperature by shaking a few drops on to the inside of your wrist – it should be lukewarm, not hot

- never use a microwave for re-warming a feed – it destroys nutrients in the milk and creates hotspots.

Sterilising

If you express milk and use a cup or bottle to feed your baby it's important that you sterilise your feeding equipment properly to make sure it is free from bacteria. You'll find all you need to know about sterilising on page 130.

This free DVD from NHS Health Scotland will give you all the information you need about breastfeeding. Ask your midwife for a copy.

from bump to
breastfeeding

breastfeeding your baby

step-by-step

Ensuring that your baby attaches properly to your breast can help to ensure a comfortable, successful feed.

Positioning

○ First of all, make sure you are comfortable – it doesn't matter if this means sitting up or lying down! Hold your baby's whole body turned towards you and tucked in very close, with her head at the level of your breast.

○ Point your nipple towards your baby's nose.

○ Allow her head to tilt back, and if she is ready to feed, her mouth will open. You can encourage this by gently rubbing your nipple across her mouth.

○ When her mouth is wide open, bring her to your breast, with her head still tilted back.

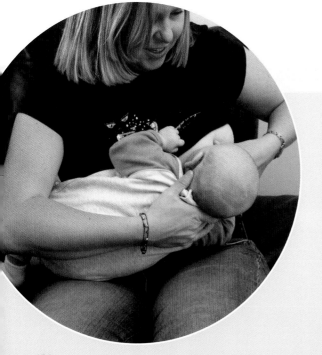

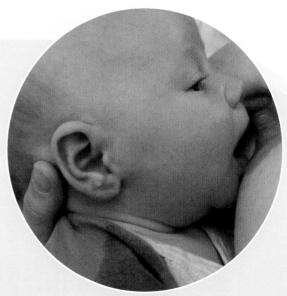

Attachment

○ Your baby needs a good mouthful of breast as well as nipple to help her feed effectively.

○ She should have a good portion of your breast below the nipple in her mouth.

Signs that your baby is well attached:

- her mouth is wide open

- her cheeks are full and rounded

- her chin is pressed into your breast

- you should be able to see more areola (the circle of darker skin surrounding your nipple) above your baby's top lip than below her bottom lip

- she begins to feed right away with rhythmic sucks and swallows that may be rapid to start with

- breastfeeding should be comfortable and pain-free

- your nipple is the same shape at the end of the feed as at the beginning.

The sleepy, reluctant feeder

All babies are different, but as a general guide, your baby should feed at least six times in 24 hours. Some babies are reluctant feeders and need encouragement to ensure that they feed often enough, and that they get enough milk. Reasons for reluctant feeding include:

- a mum who has had a lot of sedation or a long and difficult birth

- a mum who is missing feeding cues (see page 120)

- a baby who is premature or jaundiced

- on rare occasions, a baby who is unwell.

If your baby is sleepy and reluctant to feed in the first few days, you should speak to your midwife. In the meantime, you should express your milk at least six to eight times in 24 hours to build up your milk supply and prevent engorgement.

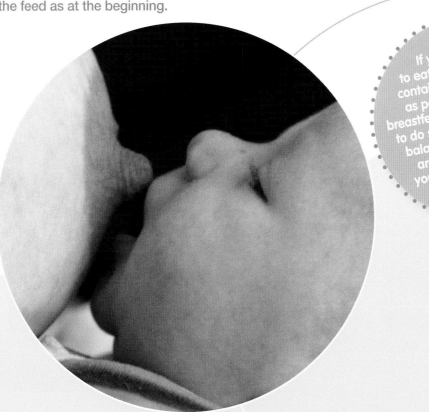

If you would like to eat peanuts or foods containing peanuts (such as peanut butter) while breastfeeding, you can choose to do so as part of a healthy balanced diet, unless you are allergic to them or your health professional advises you not to.

Formula feeding your baby

Some mums choose to bottle feed their babies with infant formula milk. This is processed, powdered cow's milk which has been treated to make it suitable for babies. There are formula milk regulations in the UK to ensure that all of the formula milks readily available in this country have the basic ingredients your baby needs.

Which formula milk should I use?

Babies should only drink formula milk, not ordinary pasteurised cow's milk, until they are a year old, although pasteurised, full-fat cow's milk can be used in cooking from six months.

First-stage formula is whey-based. It's suitable for babies until they are a year old, then they can move on to full-fat cow's milk. Second-stage or follow-on formula are both casein-based and take longer for your baby to digest, which can lead to constipation. Evidence suggests that casein-based formula is not necessary for most babies. There is no need to switch to second-stage or follow-on formula. Whey-based infant formula is fine for your baby until she switches to cow's milk.

Toddlers and young children should not have rice drinks, often known as rice milk, as a replacement for cow's milk, breast milk, or infant formula. Your midwife, health visitor/public health nurse or GP will be happy to discuss any concerns you may have with you.

Occasionally, a specialist formula based on other products can be prescribed on medical or dietetic advice. Never use soya infant formula for babies without advice from a paediatric dietician. Goat's milk infant formula is not suitable for babies as it is deficient in some basic nutrients.

There are two main sorts of formula: powdered which needs to be mixed with water, or ready made formula, which is already mixed.

Making up formula milk

When using powdered formula, it is extremely important that you follow the manufacturer's instructions on the pack regarding the correct quantity of powder and water to be mixed. Never be tempted to add extra powder as this could make your baby ill. Adding too little powder means that she will not get the nutrients and nourishment she needs.

You should always make up a fresh bottle of formula milk just before feeding. After the feed throw away any left over milk.

Feeding your baby

First of all, make sure that you are sitting comfortably and that you are supporting your baby's body and neck. She needs to be sitting slightly backwards in your arms, but not completely flat. Hold the bottle so that the teat is full, or almost full, of milk – if your baby takes in air rather than milk, this can give her a sore tummy or colic.

Always bottle feed your baby by holding her in your arms – never leave her to feed alone. Apart from being dangerous for your baby, holding her close and snuggling with her while she feeds is a wonderful opportunity to strengthen your emotional bond.

When you are bottle feeding, you may find that other people are willing to help out and take a turn. However, do make sure that you are the one to feed your baby the most. Not only does this strengthen the emotional bond between you, it also means you're best placed to notice if she's feeding properly – or to spot any potential health problems.

Winding your baby

Bottle fed babies need to be winded during and at the end of their feed to avoid wind being trapped in their tummies. You can either do this by gently sitting your baby up, supporting her under her chin and rubbing her back until she burps – or by leaning her against your shoulder and either rubbing or patting her back. As well as a burp, she might also bring up a little milk – so make sure you have a clean, dry cloth handy.

at a glance

✳ Formula milk is cow's milk which has been treated to make it suitable for babies.

✳ Babies should have formula until they are a year old then they can have ordinary full-fat cow's milk. Follow-on and toddler milks are rarely necessary.

✳ It's important to thoroughly clean and sterilise all feeding equipment such as bottles and teats.

✳ Try to bottle feed your baby yourself as much as possible rather than letting other people do it, to strengthen the emotional bond between you.

✳ Never add anything to formula milk to 'thicken' it to try to satisfy a hungry baby.

What you need for bottle feeding

Bottle feeding requires more equipment than breastfeeding. And you need to make sure you sterilise your equipment to prevent your baby getting infections and stomach upsets. You'll need the following to get you started:

- **200 ml bottles with teats and bottle covers**
- **formula milk**
- **bottle brush, teat brush**
- **sterilising equipment (such as a cold water steriliser, microwave or steam steriliser).**

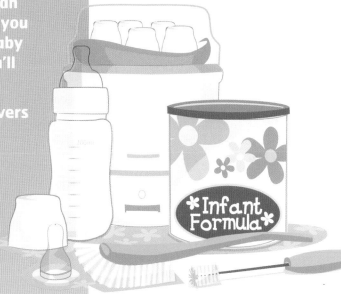

making up a feed

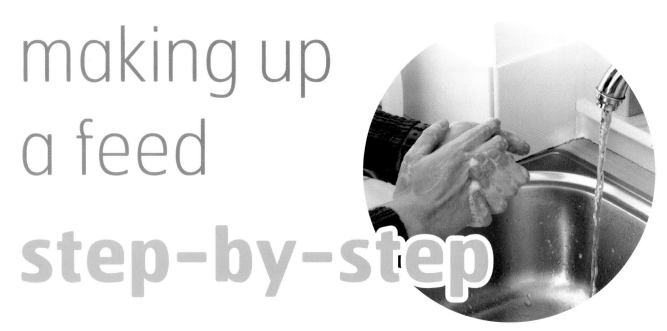

step-by-step

Powdered formula is not a sterile product and containers of formula may contain bacteria, even though they are sealed. Infections caused by bacteria in infant formula milk are very rare, but when they do happen they can be serious. There will be clear and detailed instructions on how to make up your baby's feed on the packaging of the formula you use. Make sure you follow them precisely. Here are the key things to remember.

Make sure everything's sterile

All feeding equipment must be kept clean to protect your baby against infection. It is important to wash everything after use in hot soapy water and use teat and bottle brushes to make sure all deposits are removed. If you don't use a teat brush, turn teats inside out to clean them.

All the equipment you use for feeding your baby needs to be sterilised until she is at least six months old. This includes your breast pump if you are expressing milk. Rinse all your equipment thoroughly before sterilising.

Sterilise using one of the following methods and follow manufacturer's instructions:

- a chemical sterilising solution
- steaming, in a special steam steriliser
- a sterilising unit made for the microwave oven.

Always wash your hands before removing the equipment. If you wish to rinse the equipment before using, use cooled boiled water. Store sterilising solutions safely out of reach of children.

Use boiled tap water, not bottled water

Formula feeds should be made up using cooled boiled water that is still hotter than 70°C. In practice, this means using water that has been recently boiled and left to cool in the kettle for no more than half an hour.

Use tap rather than bottled water as the content of some natural mineral waters is unsuitable for babies. However, other bottled waters are fine. You need to look for a sodium level of less than 0.2 gms per litre.

If you are abroad, you will need to use bottled water which you have boiled and allowed to cool – not tap water.

Don't over concentrate feeds

Follow the formula manufacturer's instructions about how to make up a feed. Don't feel tempted to add a little more powder if your baby is very hungry – this can make her dehydrated or constipated.

Only use fresh formula

It's important to make up a fresh bottle for each feed. This is because bacteria can multiply rapidly at room temperature and can even survive in the fridge, so storing made up formula milk for any length of time increases the chance of your baby becoming ill. Any milk left over from a feed should be thrown away. Milk left over from a feed should never be reheated.

If you need to feed your baby when you're out, boil some water, put it in a vacuum flask and take it with you. Then you can use it to prepare a feed when you need it.

Check the temperature of the milk

Test the temperature of the formula milk on the inside of your wrist. It may feel too hot, in which case put the cap over the teat and hold the bottle under cold running water to cool it down.

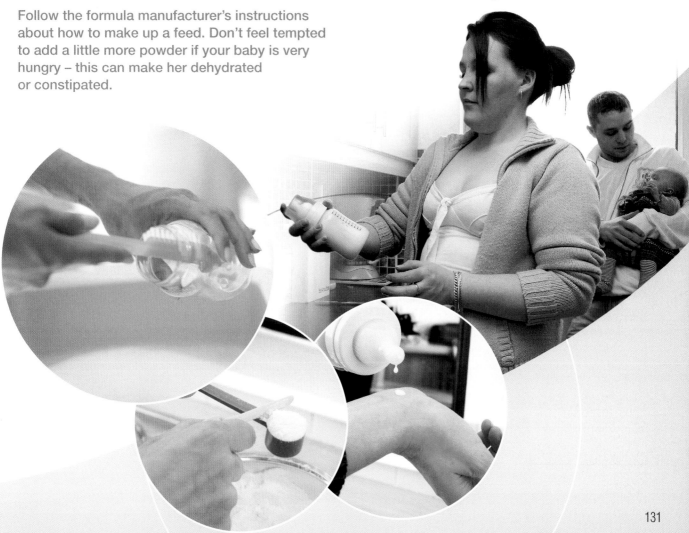

Registering the birth of your baby

The law in Scotland means that you must register the birth of your baby before she is 21 days old. You register the birth of your baby with the Registrar of Births, Deaths and Marriages. There will be a local one in your area and you can find their details through your midwife, hospital staff or in the phone book.

Parental rights and responsibilities

These give you the legal right to make decisions about your child's care, welfare, education and development. If you register the birth jointly or are married it means you share equal parental responsibilities and rights. If you do not, or are not married, only the mother assumes these rights and responsibilities. For more information please visit **www.scotland.gov.uk/familylaw**

Your midwife or hospital staff will let the Registrar of Births, Deaths and Marriages know that your baby has been born and you'll be sent a reminder letter and given an extension if you haven't registered your baby's birth within 21 days. You'll need to make an appointment with your local office and remember to take documentation with you.

If you're married...

...either of you can register the birth of your baby. You'll automatically have the same parental rights and responsibilities. You'll need to take a copy of your marriage certificate and the card you were given at the hospital with you.

If you're not married...

...the mother assumes all parental rights and responsibilities unless the father is named in the register. To do this, the father must:

- Sign the register jointly with the mother (so it means you both need to go to the Registrar's office).

- Sign a declaration which you should pick up in advance from the Registrar's office. The mother needs to sign a declaration too. The declarations are a statement that you both agree who the father of your baby is. This means the mother can register both of you as parents without the father needing to be there.

- Have a court decree declaring that he is the father and the mother can then register the birth, without the father needing to be there.

If you are not married to your baby's father, he does not have any rights regarding whether or not you choose to have your baby immunised against serious diseases *(see page 156)*.

Car safety

The law states that all children, including babies, must sit in a properly fitted child seat, suitable for their weight and height, for every journey, including the one home from hospital.

Travelling with babies

○ It is dangerous and illegal to sit a baby on your lap or in your arms on a car journey and you should never put a seatbelt around yourself and a baby. In a crash, or even a small bump, the weight of both people will be transferred through the seatbelt and could severely injure the child.

○ Rear-facing car seats should be used until your baby is able to sit up for a long time without any help.

○ Infant car seats can be used in the front or back seat and must be used in accordance with the manufacturer's instructions; however, most cars these days are fitted with airbags, and these can be dangerous to your baby if she is in the front seat. If there is an airbag on the passenger side, your baby should travel in the back.

○ Don't use a second-hand car seat unless you're absolutely sure it isn't damaged – sometimes faults can be invisible to the eye.

○ Before you buy a car seat, make sure it is the correct one for your child, and also that it will fit into your car. These are the most important aspects of choosing a seat. Additional advice can be provided by your local road safety officer or look out for the *Good Egg Guide to Car Safety,* **www.protectchild.co.uk**

○ You should learn how to use the car seat – including fitting it – before using it with your baby. You don't want to have to worry about that when you're trying to care for your baby too! Choose a shop or retailer with trained staff who will make sure you get the right seat, show you how to fit it properly, and then guide you as you fit it yourself.

○ Some hospitals hire car seats and some taxis supply them. Ask a taxi firm for this service if you ever need to use a taxi and don't have your own seat. For safety's sake, everyone in a vehicle must use a seatbelt or child seat at all times.

at a glance

✳ All children travelling in cars, including babies, must be fitted with an appropriate restraint.

✳ Never put a seatbelt around more than one person, especially a child.

✳ Never put a rear-facing car seat in the front of the car if there's an airbag on the passenger side.

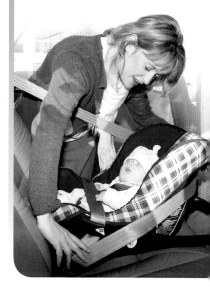

Routine care – bathing

Your baby's first baths can be quite an alarming experience. She's so small, slippery and wriggly that it's natural to be scared you'll do something wrong. You'll probably find you're being so careful that it takes you ages. That's no problem – there's no hurry – but make sure you don't let the bath water go cold!

Be prepared

In the early days you don't have to bath your baby every day. A good alternative is a quick 'top and tail' *(see page 137)*. The main thing is to make sure that the room is made free of draughts, that you have everything you need to hand – towels, fresh nappy, clean clothes – and that your baby is fully awake and ready to enjoy the experience! You must also make sure the water is not too hot.

Nooks and crannies

Some babies have lots of folds of skin – particularly round the neck, thighs and wrists. Make sure you (very gently!) clean inside these folds as they often harbour trapped milk which can not only become quite smelly, but may also cause irritation or a rash. Down below, it's important to be very gentle too – never try to pull back a baby boy's foreskin.

The stump of the umbilical cord can often become a little smelly before it finally falls off. Just let the bath water wash gently around it to remove any discharge. In about 10 days the stump will fall off, leaving a perfect little tummy button!

Fingers and toes

Baby's finger nails and toe nails can often be quite scratchy and it's important to keep them neat and trim – especially as some babies will scratch the delicate skin on their faces. It's easier to cut nails when they're soft after a bath – and when your baby is relaxed and sleepy. Use a pair of special baby nail scissors with rounded edges (never anything sharp) and don't cut too far down.

‘ **The first time I bathed my daughter I was terrified! I was sure she'd slip under the water. At first my partner used to hold her while I washed her – now I do it by myself and it's one of our nicest times together. She loves the water.** ’
Aileen, Bridge of Allan

I've heard babies can get something called cradle cap. What is it and what should I do about it?

A. Cradle cap is a scalp condition which is fairly common in babies. It shows up as scaly, greasy deposits on the scalp – rather like a particularly bad bout of dandruff. It's nothing to worry about – in fact, it's a sign that your baby's skin is growing.

You can get rid of the deposits by rubbing baby oil or vegetable oil into your baby's scalp to loosen them, then rinsing off. If the scalp becomes red or appears infected, seek advice from your midwife or health visitor/public health nurse.

Keeping your baby clean

It will probably help at first if you and your partner learn to bath your baby together — that way you can both take a turn. Pretty soon, though, you'll be a dab hand at it and wonder what the fuss was about! Lots of parents find bathing their baby is one of the nicest things about caring for them — babies usually like water and it's a chance to get to know each other too.

at a glance

✳ Your midwife or health visitor/public health nurse will be happy to answer questions.

✳ Looking after your baby can seem daunting at first but you'll get more confident as the weeks go on.

✳ Bathing her can be a challenge but you'll get the hang of it in no time!

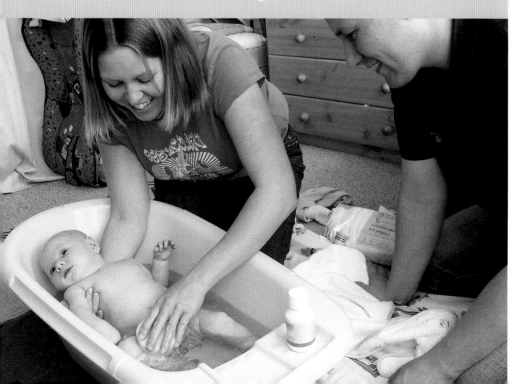

bathing your baby

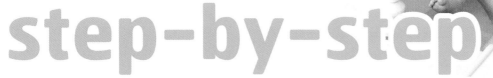

step-by-step

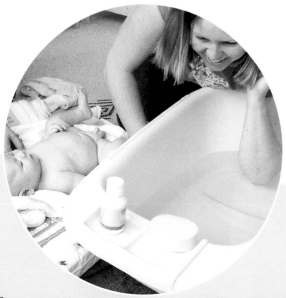

Where should I bath my baby?

Using a standard bath will require you to lean awkwardly over your baby. It can be easier in the early days to use a basin or small baby bath.

Temperature

Put the cold water in first, then the hot. Test the temperature with your elbow – it should feel comfortably warm. Don't fill the bath too high – about 15 cm will be about enough.

Lower your baby into the water on her back, supporting her head and shoulders on your hand and forearm.

Bathing

Use your free hand to wet her body and rub over the skin gently with a clean cloth. If she only has a little hair just rinse her head during the bath, pouring some water over it with a jug or your own hand.

Use plain water for newborn babies. If you like you can start using unperfumed toiletries made for babies from about four to six weeks – but use them sparingly so you don't damage your baby's developing skin.

Shampooing

Babies with longer hair may need a little drop of mild shampoo on wet hair, lathered and rinsed off. Either support your baby's head and shoulders with one hand as she lies in the bath and pour the water over with your other hand, or wrap her in a towel and hold her over the bath with one hand while you use the other hand to wash.

Drying

Dry your baby in a large, soft towel, put on her nappy and dress her.

'Top and tail' your baby

This is a quick alternative to a bath for a young baby, once or twice a day.

What you need:

- cotton wool or two soft clean cloths
- a bowl of warm water
- a fresh nappy and clean clothes if necessary
- a bin or bucket for waste.

What to do:

- first wash your own hands, then undress your baby on her back and leave her nappy on – a very new baby may be more comfortable if wrapped in a towel to stay warm
- while she is warmly wrapped up, wipe her face, neck and ears with cotton wool or a soft cloth dipped in warm water; dry with cotton wool, the other cloth or a soft towel
- wipe her underarms, then dry them

- take off your baby's nappy and, for a very new baby, wash any discharge that may have come from the stump of the umbilical cord
- wash your baby's genitals and bottom well (for girls, wipe with a clean wet cloth from front to back) then pat dry and use a protective cream if you think that your baby's skin looks red and sore
- put on a fresh nappy and dress your baby.

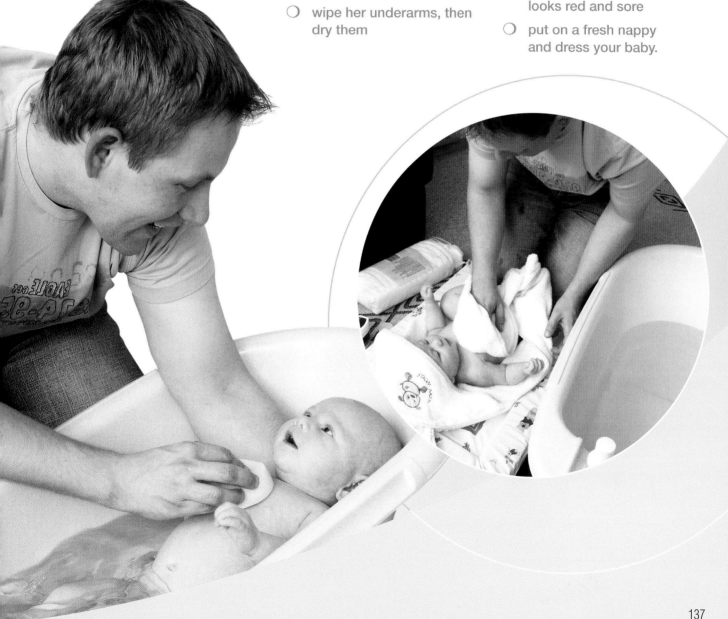

Routine care – nappies

Some parents find that disposable nappies are the most convenient option for them, while others prefer to use washable nappies. There is no doubt that washable nappies are kinder to the environment as they don't take up landfill space or take years to rot down.

Choosing nappies

You may find that a good compromise is to use throw-away liners with washable cotton nappies. The best of both worlds!

Disposable nappies

If you use disposable nappies, you'll find a wide choice of brands available, including supermarkets' own brands. Prices vary and there are options to suit most budgets. It's worthwhile trying out a few different makes to see what suits you and your baby – the most expensive option isn't necessarily the best.

Remember to dispose of soiled nappies carefully. You can buy a special nappy bin which you'll need to empty two or three times a week – or you can wrap each dirty nappy in a nappy sack and put it in the bin. It's more hygienic to put it straight in your outdoor bin.

Washable nappies

If you use washable nappies, you can wash and dry them at home yourself or, where available, use a nappy laundry service which you pay to take away dirty nappies and swap them for clean ones.

Many councils have schemes to support the use of reusable nappies. The Real Nappy Helpline on **0845 850 0606** gives callers details of their local cloth nappy contacts, whether they want to buy them to wash at home or use a laundry service. For more information on real nappies, visit **www.realnappycampaign.com**

Changing your baby's nappy

All you really need is a changing mat or clean towel and you can change your baby on the floor. Some mums prefer changing stations which allow you to stand up when you're changing your baby's nappy. If you do use a changing station, remember never to leave your baby alone on it, in case she rolls and falls.

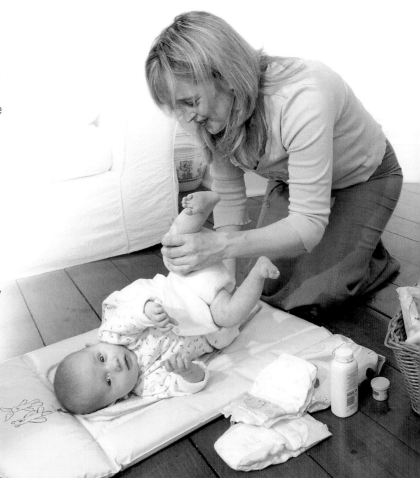

What is nappy rash and how can I prevent my baby getting it?

A. Nappy rash is quite common in babies. The symptoms are redness or soreness on and around your baby's bottom and genitals. You can help prevent this by changing dirty nappies as soon as possible and by cleaning and drying your baby's bottom carefully. You can also try leaving your baby to kick without a nappy for a short period (although this is more hazardous with baby boys as their pee can go everywhere!) If a rash seems particularly bad or infected, do speak to your health visitor/public health nurse or GP.

Washing your hands regularly can reduce bugs and other illnesses caught by both you and your child.

Time for a change?

You'll soon know when you need to change your baby's nappy – wet nappies will feel warm and full on her bottom and dirty nappies… well, you'll probably be able to smell them!

- make sure you have a clean dry nappy, a bowl of warm water, cotton wool and a small soft towel to hand

- lay your baby down on her back on the changing mat or a clean towel

- unfasten her clothes from the waist down

- unfasten and remove the dirty nappy

- hold your baby's legs and feet up

- wipe her bottom and genitals clean with cotton wool balls soaked in warm water (remember to wipe baby girls from front to back to avoid infection)

- pat her dry with the small soft towel

- apply nappy cream if she has any red or sore skin

- put on a clean nappy and wash your hands!

Hand hygiene

Washing your hands is important for both you and your baby's health. It will help to stop you and your baby from getting tummy bugs and other illnesses.

Of course, as well as taking extra care to make sure your hands are clean, with a new baby in the house you'll want to make sure that other children's hands are as clean as possible when playing with the new baby. And don't forget to be extra vigilant about wiping down surfaces and cleaning up after your pets.

Here are some examples of when you should wash your hands:

- before feeding yourself or your baby

- before making up your baby's bottle or expressing your breast milk

- after going to the toilet or changing your baby's nappy

- after touching objects that could contain germs (for example a bin or mop)

- after touching pets or anything that belongs to them (food bowls or cages).

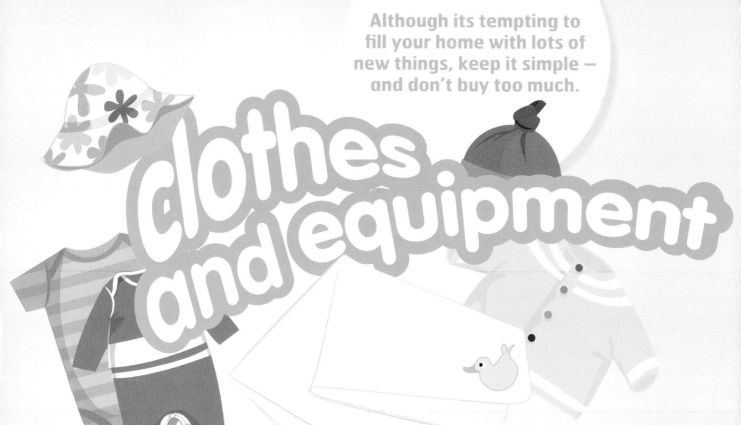

Clothes and equipment

With so many lovely baby things on offer in the shops – or online – it's all too easy to run up a huge 'wish list'. If you are lucky, you may have friends or relatives with baby clothes and equipment to hand on. This will save you a lot of money. Here's a list of the clothes and accessories that you might need for the first few weeks:

○ Five all-in-one baby grows with popper fastenings.

○ Five vests with popper fastenings.

○ Three cardigans or indoor jackets.

○ One outdoor jacket.

○ A sunhat for a summer baby; warm hat for a winter baby.

○ Pram sheets and cot sheets.

○ Cellular blankets.

○ Two towels for bathing.

○ Two washcloths for topping and tailing.

○ Six muslin or soft cotton cloths.

In addition you may want to have:

○ A cot (or crib or moses basket for the first few months).

○ A baby bath.

○ A bowl for 'topping and tailing'.

○ A changing mat.

○ Nappy sacks (if you're using disposable nappies).

○ A pram or buggy.

○ A car seat.

Babies grow much faster than you'd think. They'll grow out of their first outfits quickly and most will be too big for their baby crib by about three to six months so you'll need a full-size cot from then on.

My sister-in-law has offered me a loan of her pram. It seems in good condition and it's very kind of her but I'm worried about safety.

A. You're right to be concerned about using second-hand equipment, particularly if you don't know who it belonged to before. But in general if you know the equipment's history – and know that if it's a car seat, for instance, it hasn't been in an accident – and check it meets safety standards (*see page 133 for details of these*), it can be a good way to cut the cost of having a baby. Use your common sense and don't be afraid to say no thanks if you're worried.

Equipment for your growing baby

- Baby slings can generally be used from birth (front slings). They allow you to carry your baby close to you while leaving your arms and hands free. There's also some evidence that it can help mums and dads bond with their baby.

- By six months, you may need a high chair – make sure it has a five-point safety harness, which meets British safety standards.

- Back carriers can be used when your baby is older (from six months) and can support her own head and neck. Good retailers will allow you and your partner to try on a few models before you decide what to buy.

> Never use a second-hand mattress in your cot, crib, moses basket or pram. Always buy a new one for both hygiene and safety.

handy hints for prams

- ○ In a pram, your baby needs one or two layers of lightweight blankets on top in cold weather, a waterproof rain cover and a sheet underneath. More layers are needed in a lightweight pushchair and if the weather is exceptionally cold. If you use a fabric pushchair, or one which is low to the ground, it will be cosier with a blanket underneath your baby as well as on top.

- ○ Don't let your baby overheat. If you leave her in the pram or pushchair when you come indoors from outside (perhaps because she is asleep), take the covers off and any heavy outdoor garments.

- ○ A sun canopy or a parasol is useful in summer and essential when it's very hot. Make sure your baby is out of the direct sun at all times.

- ○ A shopping tray or basket is handy. The ones that fix underneath won't tip your pushchair over when full, if the baby starts wriggling.

Crying

All babies cry – although some babies cry a lot more than others and it's not really clear why. These babies are particularly difficult to soothe and seem unhappy a lot of the time, even if they are healthy and developing normally. Remember you can always get help if you are worried.

How to cope with a crying baby

Pick your baby up, talk to her and cuddle her as this can help with crying problems.

Parents can get exhausted and upset by a baby who never seems to stop crying. If you're getting very upset, you may find it helps to put her down somewhere safe or ask someone else to hold her and leave the room. Never, ever shake a baby, no matter how frustrated you feel – this is very dangerous. It could even be fatal.

Coping with a baby who always seems unhappy is extremely stressful, so try to make sure there's plenty of support around – ask an understanding friend to hold her for a while or ask your health visitor/public health nurse about local sources of support. Remember that some babies do cry more often than others. As you and your partner get to know your baby, you'll begin to learn what different cries mean.

Some of these steps may help:

- rocking, patting or gently rubbing your baby's back, tummy or feet (see baby massage, opposite)

- giving more frequent feeds

- carrying your baby in a sling – some like the closeness this brings

- giving your baby a warm bath

- getting a change of scene – going for a walk or a drive.

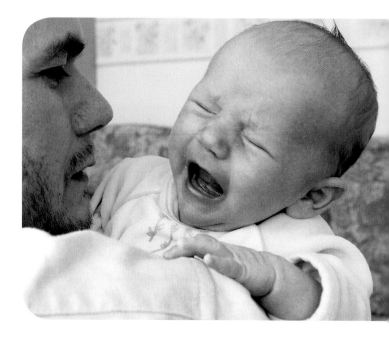

It's important to trust your instincts too so if you are worried about your baby's crying, ask your health visitor/public health nurse to check her over so that you know that everything's OK. If there's nothing wrong, you may just have to accept that this is the way your baby is. You're not doing anything wrong, it's not your fault and it happens to lots of people. Over time, she'll become more settled. There are support helplines you can call (see **Further help**, page 204).

> It seemed like nothing I could do would stop Megan crying. I felt guilty and upset as if it was my fault. I spoke to my GP who examined her and said she was OK and that some babies cried more than others. I still find it stressful but at least I know I'm not alone.
> *Elizabeth, Inverness*

Q *My baby cries a lot and my mum says its colic. What is colic and what can I do about it?*

A. Some people think that persistent crying can be caused by colic – taking in too much air when feeding causing tummy pain due to bubbles of trapped wind. Colic may also relate to poor attachment when breastfeeding or feeding too quickly from a bottle. Ask your midwife, health visitor/public health nurse or a breastfeeding counsellor for advice. You can get medicine from your GP or pharmacist. Allow three or four days for remedies to work. Gentle massage on your baby's tummy can help (see the information below on baby massage).

Baby massage

Baby massage is becoming increasingly popular and most areas now offer classes. It's just what it sounds like – gentle, soothing touching and stroking which should have benefits for you and your baby. Research suggests that skin-to-skin contact with your baby can help her thrive physically and emotionally; it can also help you become more confident as a parent. You can start when your baby is about six weeks old – but don't do anything your baby doesn't like.

Depending on the part of Scotland you live in, your NHS Board may offer you the play@home books. The first in the series offers a very good section on baby massage with useful diagrams. Your midwife or health visitor/public health nurse can give you details of baby massage classes in your area.

at a glance

❋ All babies cry – some more than others.

❋ A baby who cries constantly can be exhausting and worrying for parents.

❋ If you are concerned about your baby's crying, trust your instincts and seek help.

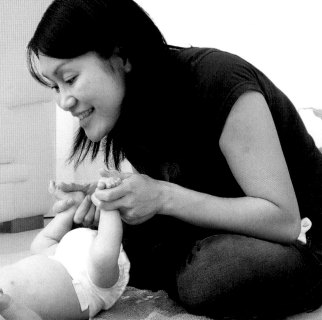

Getting a good night's sleep

A full night's sleep is one of the things that many new parents miss most after their baby is born. Newborn babies only sleep for a few hours at a time and it's normal for them to need to be fed during the night.

If your baby is unwell, get medical advice.

Some tips for a good night's sleep

It's not realistic to expect your baby to sleep several times a day and wake only for feeds and to smile and coo. Some babies may behave like this but most don't. As long as you understand this, you can prepare for it – and look forward to the time when she sleeps through the night!

Back to sleep

To keep your baby safe when she is sleeping always put her to sleep on her back. This decreases the risk of cot death (or sudden infant death syndrome).

Feet to foot

When you put your baby down in her moses basket, cradle or cot to sleep, always position her at the bottom – that is, with her feet at the foot of her cot – not with her head at the top. That way, she can't wriggle down and get caught under her blankets.

Blankets and covers

For newborn babies, cellular blankets (the ones the hospital uses) are the best. They help keep your baby's temperature regular – neither too hot nor too cold – and they're light. Baby duvets, fleece blankets and cot bumpers are not recommended for newborn babies.

Room temperature

The ideal temperature for a baby's room is between 16°C and 20°C. At this temperature, your baby will only need one or two layers of cellular blanket to keep her snug all night long. Make sure that her room is free from draughts.

Lighting and music

You might find that a night light is comforting in a baby's room – it also means that you won't trip over in the dark when you go in to check on her. For some babies, a gentle lullaby as she's going off to sleep is soothing and helps to create an association with a sleep routine. You can either sing yourself – or you might prefer a musical box or toy instead, depending on your musical skills!

Don't forget yourself

When you can, take time to have a relaxing bath before bed. Ask your partner, or a friend to take over for an hour. You might still only get four hours' sleep before you're up for another feed, but at least you've had a little 'me time'!

Plagiocephaly

You may have heard about babies developing a persistent flat spot, either at the back of or on one side of the head. This is known as plagiocephaly – it is cosmetic and will not affect your baby's brain. It sometimes happens when babies lie in the same position for long periods. To help avoid this, make sure your baby has supervised 'playtime' on her tummy but never let her fall asleep like this. If you are worried and want more information ask your midwife or health visitor/public health nurse.

You should receive a copy of the leaflet *Protect your baby's natural headshape: tummy time to play, back to sleep* either before or shortly after the birth of your baby. And you can find more information at **www.scotland.gov.uk/ resource/doc/170857/0047857.pdf**

Q *How much sleep is normal for my baby?*

A. Some babies sleep more than others – there's no normal amount of sleep. All babies have days when they want to sleep more and days when they are more wakeful than usual. New babies sleep a lot – this may be as much as 18 hours a day for the first month or so. However, they will rarely sleep for more than a few hours at a time. A baby who seems unusually sleepy may be unwell, you should trust your instincts and get medical advice if you are worried.

Safe sleeping

The safest place for your baby to sleep is feet to foot (with her feet at the foot of the cot) in a cot in your room for the first six months. While it's lovely to have your baby with you for a cuddle or a feed, it's safest to put your baby back in her cot before you go back to sleep. Risks associated with bed sharing are increased if you or your partner smoke, have recently drunk alcohol, have taken medication or drugs that could make you sleepy, or are very tired.

at a glance

✳ New babies only sleep for a few hours at a time.

✳ It's normal for babies to be hungry during the night.

✳ Babies' sleeping habits change as they grow.

It's very dangerous for you or anyone else to fall asleep with a baby in a sofa or armchair.

reducing the risk of cot death

Cot death, or sudden infant death syndrome, claims less than 50 infants a year in Scotland. It's rare, and we don't yet know what causes it. We do know, however, that there are ways of reducing the risks.

- Always place your baby on her back to sleep.
- Keep your baby away from cigarette smoke – and remember that it can linger on clothes too.

- Don't let anyone smoke in a room where your baby is going to sleep.
- Don't fall asleep with a small baby in bed or on a sofa or armchair.
- Place your baby with her feet at the foot of her cot so she can't wriggle underneath her blankets.
- Make sure your baby doesn't get too hot or cold. Check her temperature by feeling her stomach or the back of her neck – don't go by her hands and feet as they will often feel cold.

Ask your health professional for a copy of the leaflet *Reduce the risk of Cot Death.*

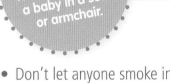

Looking after yourself

Most new parents say they can't believe how utterly exhausted they feel once they start looking after a new baby. It really is a life-changing experience. That is enough to get used to, but on top of it all you're probably not getting much sleep!

Coping with tiredness

Sheer exhaustion can make it harder to cope, especially when things aren't going exactly as you planned or hoped, but it's important to remember that this is normal and it will pass. If it doesn't *(see **Baby blues**, page 113 and **Postnatal depression**, pages 158–163)* talk to your midwife, health visitor/public health nurse or GP.

If you find yourself getting really tired, try and have a little nap during the day when your baby does.

Staying active

It's important to build some form of exercise into your day. Try to do it gradually at first by getting into the habit of taking your baby out in the pram, buggy or sling at least once a day. Take the stairs, not the lift and walk to the shops instead of getting in the car. It's good exercise for you and gets you out of the house. A change of scene can often calm your baby if she is crying and will help you feel better too.

If you were quite fit before giving birth, then you'll want to know how long to wait before exercising again. There's no hard and fast rule. You will need to wait until the discharge (lochia) has stopped before going swimming. Or wait until your stitches have gone before attempting a high impact fitness class. But you'll probably know yourself when you're up to it and, if in doubt, ask your health visitor/public health nurse.

> I'm trying to get out with the pram. Everyone in the village is always so pleased to see the baby – it gives me a real lift.
>
> *Ellen, Perthshire*

Out and about

○ **Physical activity is good for you and your baby.**

○ **Going for walks with your baby can help develop a close bond.**

○ **Aim to gradually build up to 30 minutes of moderate physical activity on most days of the week. Brisk walking, swimming and playing with your baby are ideal and will help give you more energy.**

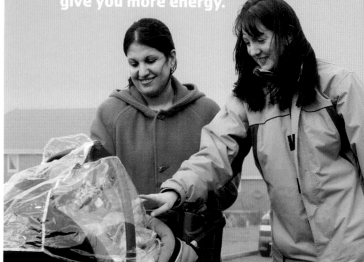

Pelvic floor exercises

Pelvic floor muscles are important because they help prevent stress incontinence (when you leak a few drops of urine when you cough, laugh or run). It's very common to feel you have no control over these muscles for a couple of days – maybe weeks – after the birth.

Ideally you'll have been doing pelvic floor exercises throughout your pregnancy. Now the more often you do the exercises, the better; and it's good to make them part of your daily routine. You'll be taught how to do them by a midwife or physiotherapist. Remember you can do them anywhere and no one will notice! You should aim to do them several times a day.

If your pelvic floor muscles are weak you may find exercising them quite difficult at first. With frequent practise though, you will soon improve. If you continue to have problems, mention it to your GP at your postnatal check and ask to be referred to a physiotherapist.

how to do the exercises

Try to use your pelvic floor muscles during everyday tasks such as getting out of bed.

Exercise 1 – Slow contractions

- Imagine you are trying to stop yourself passing wind.
- At the same time, imagine that you are trying to stop the flow of urine.
- It will feel like squeezing shut and lifting the back and front passages.
- Start by trying to hold for three seconds. Rest for five seconds then repeat the exercise.
- Build up to holding for 10 seconds. Repeat up to 10 times. Do five sets per day.

Once you are able to hold for five seconds and repeat at least five times, then you can add exercise 2.

Exercise 2 – Fast contractions

- Squeeze and lift as in exercise 1.
- Let go straight away.
- Repeat 10 times.

Don't

- tighten your buttocks
- hold your breath
- squeeze your thighs together.

Don't stop the flow of urine midstream as an exercise as it may cause incomplete bladder emptying and increase the risk of infection.

Relationships

Having a baby is a time of great change. While all attention (including yours!) may be on the baby, you need to feel that you are still 'you'. Your own needs at this time are really important – not least because you'll feel more confident as a parent if you're feeling happy in yourself.

You and your family

Offers of help can be welcome and some should certainly be accepted. However, constant visitors and advice you don't want are not so welcome. Don't feel you have to entertain people – let them make their own cup of tea and bring their own biscuits. And if it's too tiring to see someone, don't be afraid to ask them to arrange to come another time. 'Always phone first' is a good rule. Partners can be good gatekeepers by explaining that you're just too tired. Grandparents can help keep people away too but they should remember that there are times when you won't want to see them either!

You and your partner

In theory, having a baby should be a joyous time which brings you and your partner closer. In fact, it can put a real strain on even the best relationships. You can both be tired, can feel your world has been turned upside down (it has!) and the father in particular can feel 'shut out' by the new arrival. Your sex life may well suffer – and that can put pressure on you both *(see page 150)*. Learning to look after the baby together is good for a relationship. Mums should encourage partners to share the baby care and, remember, there's more than one right way to do most things.

But the most important thing is to keep talking to each other. Try to spend some time alone as a couple, even if it's just a walk for half an hour or an undisturbed meal while someone else looks after your baby.

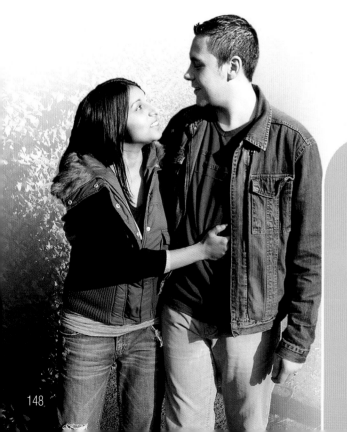

Time to yourself and adult conversation are often the most important things to new mums. If people offer to help, let them. Sometimes people will offer to bring round meals, do a bit of shopping for you or even (if you're really lucky) do the cleaning. Say yes and, remember, they'll feel good about being able to help so actually you're doing them the favour! And, if they don't offer, don't be afraid to ask.

> My boyfriend left me when I was pregnant and doesn't want to know. I knew it would be hard doing this on my own but I hadn't realised how hard. I know it's awful and I really love my baby but sometimes I just wish I could go out with my pals like I used to.
>
> *Kayleigh, Inverness*

Making friends

Having a baby can be a good way to make new friends – and chances are, you'll need them. However much you think having a baby won't change anything, it may well affect your friendships with those who don't have babies (and who still want to go out clubbing every weekend!).

Most areas will have groups of other parents that are good for support and friendship. Some organisations have coffee groups, drop-in centres or baby and toddler clubs. It can be hard to break into these networks, especially if you're a bit shy. You could ask someone you already know if they'll come with you for the first few times until you get to know other people there. Ask your health visitor/public health nurse for advice and details of groups.

If you're on your own

Try to organise as much support as possible from your family and friends. Remember it's important to make time for you as well as for the baby. There are groups that can help when it all seems too much. Ask your health visitor/public health nurse or contact groups such as Gingerbread Scotland or One Parent Families Scotland (see **Further help** page 205).

> My partner and I can't believe how lucky we are to have our lovely baby. Every time we look at him we feel blessed.
>
> *Jim, Aberdeen*

at a glance

✳ Don't be too proud to accept help.

✳ Taking care of yourself and your needs will help you become a confident parent.

✳ Try to spend some time alone with your partner and keep lines of communication open.

✳ Don't feel you have to see people if you're too tired – and that includes your new baby's grandparents.

✳ Suggest people should always phone first – and don't be too polite to say 'no'.

✳ Friendships are an important source of support and help you feel you're still 'you'.

✳ Your health visitor/ public health nurse can put you in touch with groups of other parents.

✳ If you're on your own, family and friends can offer vital support and your health visitor/public health nurse can put you in touch with other places where you can get help.

Sex and contraception

Shortly after giving birth you may feel like you'll never want to have sex again! But at some point, you probably will, so it's good to be prepared for how you might be feeling physically and emotionally – and to consider what form of contraception you may want to use.

It's OK to wait

Physically, there's no real reason why you shouldn't make love as soon as your vaginal discharge (lochia) has cleared up (usually after about four weeks), and any cut or tear in your perineum has healed. Before that, there's a risk of infection.

In practice, many couples wait longer than that. Either of you may be too tired for sex. The new mum may feel a bit bruised from the birth (physically and emotionally) and may want to wait a while. There's no right or wrong – it's up to you when you feel ready – different people want to resume their sex life at different points.

Keep talking

This can be a tough time for relationships. Try to spend some time together (to remind yourselves why you like each other) and, most importantly, keep talking to each other about how you feel. Couples should make it clear that they're not rejecting each other!

Taking your time

Remember there are other ways of being close that don't involve penetrative sex. And cuddling is almost always welcome! When you do feel the time is right, don't be surprised if it feels a bit strange and different. Your muscles can take several months to get back to normal. Remember too that you'll both probably be a bit nervous, so use some lubrication and don't rush it.

Sometimes you can feel too 'dry' for sex after childbirth and vaginal dryness caused by low oestrogen levels during breastfeeding can make sexual intercourse uncomfortable. A water-based lubricant such as KY Jelly can help and won't damage condoms or diaphragms. Don't use oil-based lubricants such as Vaseline as they can damage these forms of contraception. If sex actually hurts, talk to your GP as you may have an infection.

Is breastfeeding a form of contraception?

A. Some people believe they can't get pregnant while breastfeeding. The truth is that you can only rely on breastfeeding as a contraceptive in very controlled and specific circumstances. For example, it's only suitable for women who are exclusively breastfeeding – often and including during the night – and who never give bottles or any solid food at all. Also, periods should not have returned and the baby must be under six months old.

If you want to use this method of contraception, which is known as lactational amenorrhoea, talk to a GP first. Even using this method properly is no guarantee against pregnancy.

Using contraception

You should start using your chosen method of contraception within four weeks of the birth if you don't want to become pregnant again. Health professionals bring up the issue now so that you can think about it before it becomes more pressing. It may be that the method of contraception you used before you became pregnant may not be the most suitable one now.

The pill

If you're breastfeeding, it's recommended that you avoid the combined pill (types with both oestrogen and progesterone) as the oestrogen will reduce the amount of milk you produce. The mini-pill (progesterone only) is thought to be more suitable, but can have side-effects. You also need to be a lot stricter about making sure you take it at the same time every day. However, there is a new type of progesterone-only pill which has a twelve hour missed-pill window.

Family planning experts may be able to suggest other methods, such as progesterone implants or an injection, which mean you don't have to remember to take the pill every day.

The diaphram, cap or IUD

If you use a diaphragm or cap, you need to get it checked to make sure it still fits as the size and shape of the cervix can change during birth. Some women decide to use IUD (intrauterine device) contraception which is inserted in the womb. Usually this can't be fitted until two to three months after the birth, so other methods would have to be used in the meantime.

Condoms

The condom is the simplest choice of contraception for many women and can be used with other forms of birth control. Condoms are available free from family planning clinics and many GP surgeries.

at a glance

✳ Sex may be the last thing on your mind but it's important to think about contraception now.

✳ Some people take longer than others to want to have sex again.

✳ The important thing is to keep talking to your partner so that neither of you feels rejected.

your growing baby

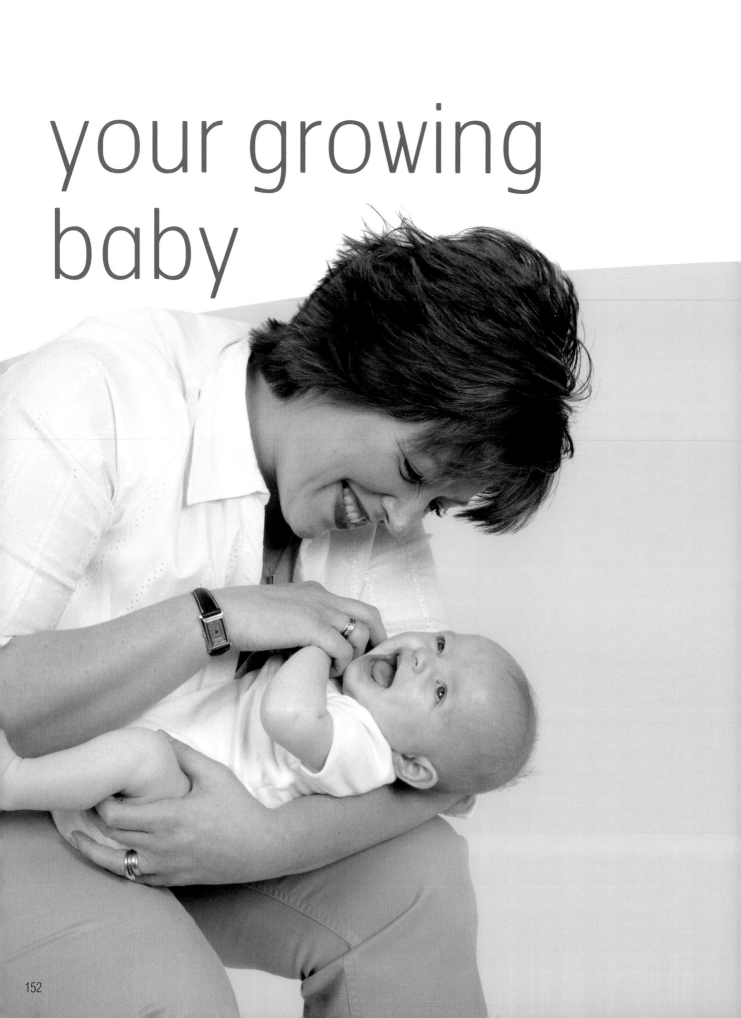

Section 4

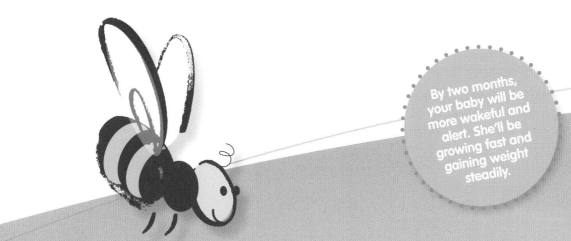

What you can expect at

1–2 months

Now that your baby is a month old, you will be beginning to get to know her, and your life together may have started to settle into some kind of pattern. It's still early days to expect to be in a regular routine, but this will emerge over the coming weeks and months.

Such a lot happens during your baby's first two months. Most babies reach certain milestones at around about the same age – but infant development isn't an exact science.

Your baby will grow and develop at her own unique pace. This depends on many factors including genetics and environment as well as your baby's temperament and her medical history.

Even at this early stage, there are many things you can do to help her develop. Talk to your baby as much as possible. Read to her, tell her stories and nursery rhymes, describe what you are doing as you go about your day. This early communication is critical to her speech and language development – and she'll love hearing the sound of your voice!

The first two months can be both magical and worrying – in equal measures! You probably have lots of questions to ask about your baby – and your skills as a new mum. 'Is she feeding enough?' 'Is she sleeping too much?' 'Am I being a good parent?' Relax, it's natural to have these concerns – and it shows that you care. But remember, if you do have any worries at all, or even just want to chat things through, speak to your health visitor/public health nurse who'll be happy to help you.

at **1–2** months your baby may be able to...

- smile on purpose, blow bubbles and coo when you talk or gently play together – newborn babies are sensitive to the way you hold, rock and feed them

- mimic your facial expressions – stick your tongue out or make funny faces and see if she copies you

- reach for you when she needs attention, security or comfort

- stretch and kick more vigorously as the weeks go by

- respond to the sound of your voice

- respond to loud noises by blinking, startling, frowning or waking from a light sleep

- move her limbs more, or slows down her sucking rhythm, when she hears familiar household noises like footsteps or running bath water

- begin to face straight ahead while lying on her back and lift her head while lying on her tummy – remember that her head will be wobbly at first so it will be several weeks before she is able to do this.

six-week postnatal check

Around six weeks after the birth, you'll be asked to see your GP or a doctor. This is routine and is meant to make sure you're in good health and that any problems can be dealt with. Your baby will be given a health check around this stage to ensure everything is alright.

This also gives you a chance to ask any questions and to talk about how you're feeling. The subject of contraception may be raised, although it might have been discussed with you already, shortly after your baby was born (see **Sex and contraception**, page 150).

Your baby's **immunisations**

If you have questions, speak to your health visitor/public health nurse, GP or practice nurse.

Immunisation is the safest and most effective way of protecting your baby against some serious diseases. Your baby will be offered her first immunisations when she is two months old.

What is immunisation?

Immunisation protects us from serious diseases. Once we have been immunised our bodies are better able to fight diseases we come in contact with.

Vaccines and immunity

Breastfeeding will certainly boost your baby's immune system and help protect against infections such as the common cold and tummy upsets but it does not protect against major childhood diseases.

Some babies have temporary side-effects such as redness and swelling where they have had the injection or may feel a bit irritable and unwell and have a fever. Your health visitor/public health nurse or GP may suggest you give your baby a dose of infant paracetamol or ibuprofen liquid if she gets a fever. From two months you can give a single 2.5 ml dose of paracetamol, and from three months a single 2.5 ml dose of infant ibuprofen. Read the instructions on the bottle carefully.

Immunisation when your baby is unwell

If your baby has a minor illness without a fever, such as a cold, she can have her immunisations as normal. However if your baby is ill with a fever, delay the immunisation until she has recovered. This is to avoid the fever being associated with the vaccine, or the vaccine increasing the fever. If your baby has a bleeding disorder or has had a fit not associated with fever, she can receive immunisations, but may need additional care, so speak to your health visitor/public health nurse or practice nurse first.

Immunisation and premature babies

Premature babies may be at a greater risk of infection. They should be immunised according to the recommended schedule from two months after birth, regardless of how premature they were.

Your immunisation appointment

You will be sent an appointment by your GP surgery when it's time to bring your baby in for her immunisations. The nurse or GP will explain the process, ask about any known allergies your baby has, and answer any questions you have. The vaccine is then injected into the muscle of your baby's thigh.

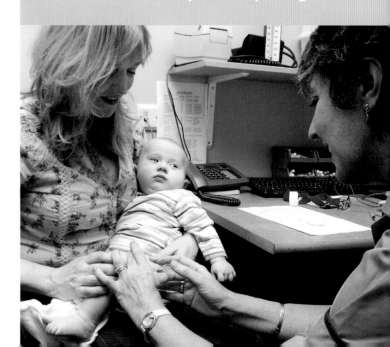

Each vaccination is given as a single injection into the thigh muscle.

Routine Childhood Immunisation Programme

When to immunise	Disease protected against	Vaccine given
2 months old	• Diphtheria, tetanus, pertussis (whooping cough), polio and Haemophilus influenzae type b (Hib) • Pneumococcal infection	• DTaP/IPV/Hib • Pneumococcal conjugate vaccine (PCV)
3 months old	• Diphtheria, tetanus, pertussis (whooping cough), polio and Haemophilus influenzae type b (Hib) • Meningococcal C (Men C)	• DTaP/IPV/Hib • Men C
4 months old	• Diphtheria, tetanus, pertussis (whooping cough), polio and Haemophilus influenzae type b (Hib) • Meningococcal C (Men C) • Pneumococcal infection	• DTaP/IPV/Hib • Men C • PCV
Around 12 months old	• Haemophilus influenzae type b (Hib) and meningococcal C (Men C)	• Hib/Men C
Around 13 months old	• Measles, mumps and rubella (German measles) • Pneumococcal infection	• MMR • PCV

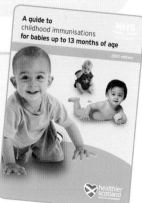

A guide to childhood immunisations for babies up to 13 months of age

2010 edition

For more information, see the booklet *A guide to childhood immunisation for babies up to 13 months of age*, which should be available from your GP surgery.

See also www.healthscotland.com

Postnatal depression (PND)

PND is more common than you might think – affecting between 10–20% of new mums. It can hit you days, weeks or months after the birth of your baby. But help is at hand, and you're not alone. Remember that although PND can be a bewildering and frightening experience, with the right support and treatment, you will be able to make a full recovery.

Symptoms of PND

Post natal depression commonly appears as overwhelmingly negative feelings – of loneliness and guilt, anxiety and irritability, tearfulness and exhaustion, anger and frustration. It may affect your appetite, your sleep patterns, your interest in sex and your concentration. For some women the feelings are quite mild, for others they are overwhelming.

Help is available

PND varies from woman to woman – as do its causes, and its treatment. But for every woman there is treatment and support available – and the sooner you seek help, the sooner you'll be back to feeling like yourself again.

What causes PND?

Medical experts don't completely understand what causes PND, but it is clear that different factors can trigger PND in different women. These can range from stressful events and circumstances in your life to the sheer pressures and expectations of parenthood – particularly if your new baby is very demanding or if you don't feel an immediate bond with her. For some women, these feelings can just come out of the blue – and that in itself is extremely stressful and upsetting.

Risk factors and triggers for PND

Evidence suggests that risk factors for developing PND include a personal or family history of mental health problems, stressful experiences in your life, recent difficult events or situations, domestic abuse or substance abuse. Mums are therefore encouraged to share that information with their midwife or GP before their baby is born, so that signs of PND can be spotted early on.

For some women, a poor birthing experience – or giving birth to a premature baby, or a baby with a health problem or disability – can trigger PND. For other women, lack of support from a partner, friends or family can be the cause, as can anxieties about your finances, housing or lifestyle.

There is no hard medical evidence to support the claim that hormonal changes in your body after the birth can cause PND, although for some women, this may be a factor. It is important to remember that PND is very different from the hormonal 'swing' of the baby blues *(see page 113)* and doesn't pass after a few days. Some women can even experience antenatal depression during their pregnancy.

> I had thought I would love my baby straight away – isn't that what you're supposed to feel? But all I felt was tired and sore. I wanted people to pay some attention to me – and I felt guilty for thinking like that.
>
> *Marina, Glasgow*

How PND might make you feel

PND can be exhausting and frightening. Feelings of loneliness and guilt, tearfulness and frustration, irritability and anxiety are all common. You may feel worried and pessimistic about the future or overly concerned about your baby's health.

Feeling lonely

For many new mums, it's not unusual to feel lonely after the birth of your baby – particularly if you've given up work or are no longer able to go out shopping or on nights out with your friends. And if you don't have a partner, or close friends and family around you on a regular basis, then it's especially tough.

Feeling guilty

Society seems to expect all new mums to be delighted when their baby is born and to fall naturally into motherhood. Often, this just isn't the case and if you don't bond with your baby straight away *(see page 110)* you might feel guilty as a result. Guilt can sometimes trigger depression – as well as be a symptom of it.

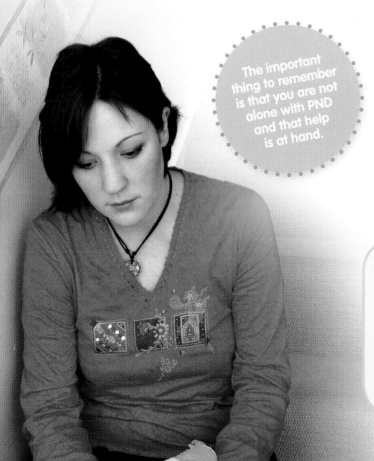

The important thing to remember is that you are not alone with PND and that help is at hand.

Feeling down

Sometimes, even when things seem to be going really well, PND can just come right out of the blue. This can be confusing and upsetting. Feeling down for no reason may make you feel anxious and guilty – and that can make your PND worse. It's a vicious circle.

Puerperal psychosis

Very rarely, mothers can suffer from a condition called puerperal psychosis, a severe mental illness which is different from PND.

Puerperal psychosis affects one to two out of 1,000 new mums and can involve severe mood changes, loss of touch with reality, and hallucinations. Often it begins within a few days of childbirth and almost always within the first three months. It is most likely to be caused by the hormone changes that occur shortly after childbirth. The risk of puerperal psychosis is much higher if you have had a similar illness before, or if you, or a member of your family, suffers from a manic-depressive disorder (such as bipolar affective disorder). It's important to be aware of this as, for women at high risk, treatments are available which can lower the risk or even prevent the illness completely.

Unlike PND, where the symptoms can be hidden, with puerperal psychosis you are usually obviously ill and need psychiatric help, possibly in hospital. Here you'll be in the right surroundings, supported by trained staff, who'll help you and your baby get the care you need.

There's more information in NHS Health Scotland's *Talking about postnatal depression* leaflet available from your midwife, health visitor/ public health nurse or GP.

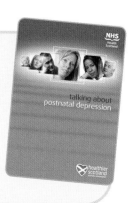

Getting help with PND

Leaving PND untreated can be harmful as it can affect all your relationships – in particular, how you bond with your baby. The first step to getting better is to talk about how you're feeling.

You're not alone

Some mums with PND try to hide it because they think they should be coping and worry about admitting that they're finding it tough. You might also worry that your baby will be taken away from you. That won't happen. In fact, every effort is made to keep mum and baby together. There are a number of ways in which you'll both be helped and supported.

Talk about it

Talk to your midwife, health visitor/public health nurse or GP (you may want to talk to your partner, friend or a member of your family first). They all have a wealth of experience in helping new mums with PND and the earlier you open up to them, the sooner you'll be on the road to recovery.

Counselling and psychotherapy

For most women with PND, the best treatment is counselling and support. This begins with your health visitor or public health nurse who can listen to you, and discuss your feelings with you. This may be enough, or you may decide together that more in-depth counselling or therapy is required. If so, that will be arranged for you.

Self help

Many women find that self help groups, which offer support and counselling with input from an experienced counsellor, are a great help. You can share your feelings with other mums who are dealing with PND, or who have gone through it in the past. Finding out that you are not alone and realising that other people know how you are feeling is often the first step to getting better. Your health visitor/public health nurse will be able to put you in touch with a local group or service.

Medical treatment

Although most mums with PND will not need anti-depressants, you and your GP may decide that this is the best course of action for you – and it may go hand-in-hand with counselling. If you are breastfeeding, your GP will prescribe a drug which will not affect your baby. Anti-depressants may be prescribed for up to a year, and although this seems like a long time, it's important that you don't stop taking them without consulting your GP, even if you start to feel better. These drugs can take two to four weeks before they begin to take effect and they need to be taken for up to six months after you've started to feel better. This can help to prevent your depression from recurring.

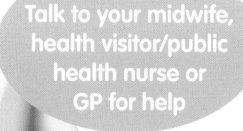

Talk to your midwife, health visitor/public health nurse or GP for help

do you have pnd?

- Do you wake up every morning feeling exhausted and as though you haven't had any sleep?
- Do you find it hard to concentrate or to organise even the simplest of things?
- Do you feel a failure?
- Do you find yourself crying or feeling tearful at small things or for no reason at all?
- Do you sometimes feel numb as if nothing is really 'reaching' you?

- Is it hard, if not impossible, to see 'the funny side' of things?
- Can you only be yourself with your partner or closest friend and sometimes not even then?
- Do you find yourself worrying constantly about your baby and family?

If you answered yes to any of these and the symptoms have gone on for more than a few days, then you may have PND.

Overcoming postnatal depression together

Postnatal depression can affect the whole family, not just the new mum. Your partner, family and friends can play a huge role in supporting you if you suffer from PND. There are also various ways in which you can help yourself too – alongside any treatment you're getting.

Postnatal depression and your partner

Your partner can have a particularly important role to play in your recovery, because sometimes they are the only person you can be yourself with.

Your partner can be a great source of support, love and understanding and can encourage you to seek help as well as be with you when you speak to your health visitor/public health nurse, midwife or GP. Chances are they may even be better at remembering what is said in a consultation – or help by writing things down that you want to say. Remember that they want to help because they care about you and your baby – not because they think you're a failure.

However, partners can also bear the brunt of your tears, anger and distress. This can be exhausting and upsetting to live with and some partners may feel angry, excluded or even overwhelmed at this time.

Research has shown that men whose partners have PND are at a higher risk of depression themselves, so remember that your GP can help your partner too.

Look after yourself

At a time when everyone's focus is on your new baby, it's all too easy to lose sight of your own needs. Just getting a little 'me' time can give you some much needed breathing space! So, take up any offers of help around the house or with your baby and try and do some of the following things for yourself:

- indulge in a treat or meet up with some friends for coffee

- try and put your feet up when your baby's asleep

- get into a night-time routine – have a bath, a hot drink and read for a while

- do some exercise – even just a short walk can make you feel physically better and that can make you feel emotionally better too

- make sure you eat regular, nutritious meals, rather than quick-fix snacks

- express your feelings – talk to someone you trust, or write it all down.

'I tried to be a good dad and help my partner with the baby. But everything I did was wrong and she always criticised me. I realised we needed help and our GP diagnosed PND. It was tough, but with treatment my partner was soon on the mend and we're a good family again. '

Sanjay, Dundee

How partners, family or friends can help

Partners can play a crucial role in spotting the signs of PND and persuading the affected mum to seek help. So if you're close to someone and think she may be suffering, refer to the questions on page 161 on her behalf and encourage her to seek help, for your and the baby's sake, as well as hers.

○ **Getting plenty of rest is important for all new mums. Offer to look after the baby so that she can have a good rest, ideally in the middle of the day.**

○ **Help round the house — cooking, cleaning or laundry.**

○ **Encourage her to look after herself by eating regularly, drinking plenty of water and taking a break now and then.**

○ **Take the baby out for a walk in the pram for a couple of hours, pick up essentials from the supermarket, make up a sandwich for lunch time and leave it in the fridge with some other snacks.**

○ **Be prepared to listen, encourage her to seek help from her GP, health visitor/public health nurse or midwife and remember that it will pass.**

at a glance

✳ Postnatal depression (PND) is common, and affects up to 20% of new mums.

✳ Women with PND need lots of support and understanding.

✳ PND is treatable — your health visitor/ public health nurse, GP or midwife can help.

✳ Don't try and be supermum — accept help when it's offered and remember to look after yourself.

✳ Involve your partner, family and friends in your recovery — you're not alone, so don't shut them out.

✳ Look after yourself — find 'me' time and try and do things you enjoy.

✳ Remember that you will get better.

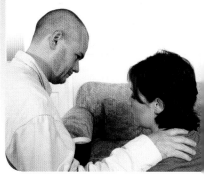

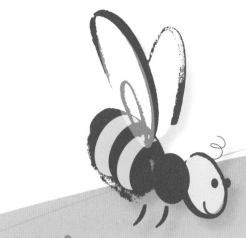

What you can expect at
3–4 months

Your baby will have come a long way in the last three months and many parents find that this is a hugely enjoyable time. You have more confidence as a parent, and your baby is becoming more sociable and enjoys being with you. You'll probably also have learned enough about her personality and behaviour to understand what she wants… most of the time!

Your baby will be able to recognise you now, as well as a couple of other familiar faces. You'll notice that she is able to make more noises and louder sounds and chuckles when she interacts with people.

Around now is a good time to think about an evening routine. If you follow a similar pattern each night, you'll find that your baby will start to show excitement as she knows what to expect – for example she'll know that after her bath she gets a feed and a story before going to bed. Some babies even start to sleep through the night at this point… but most don't!

at **3–4** months your baby may be able to...

○ keep her head up almost straight when she's in a sitting position (make sure she's supported) and her back is straighter than before

○ wave and kick more forcefully – make sure there's nothing dangerous such as hot drinks for her to kick over

○ open her fingers and bring her hands together

○ wriggle; so there's a risk she may fall out of your arms, off the bed or other high surfaces *(see page 187)*

○ follow sounds – try ringing a little bell behind her and moving it around

○ 'stand' on your lap with your help and, by four months, may be starting to take some of her own weight, but only when she's supported

○ support her head and chest with her arms when lying on her stomach

○ open and shut her hands and start to use her hands and eyes to coordinate

○ begin to babble and imitate some sounds

○ enjoy playing with other people.

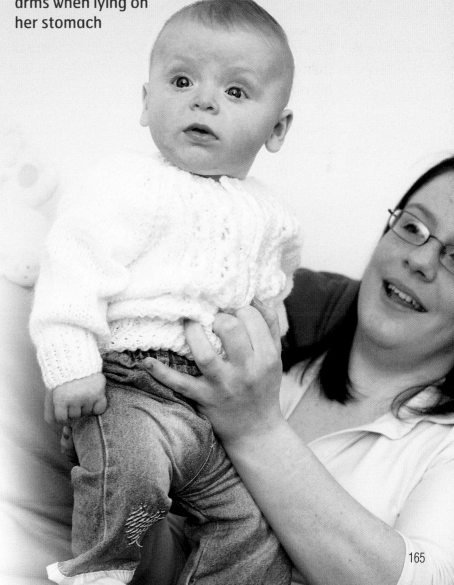

Playing with your baby at **3–4 months**

This is the time when mums and dads can really get to know their baby. It's very important to chat to her as much as possible. Although she doesn't understand what you're saying, she can hear the patterns of your speech and is learning how to communicate. It's important to have 'face-to-face' time with your baby to help these social and communication skills develop. She's also learning that if she responds to attention she'll get more of it!

Play ideas

From about three months, she can hold things and she will soon start to develop hand-eye coordination – that means she can hold something like a rattle and look at it too. Here are some play ideas. It helps to turn off the TV first!

- Sing songs and see if she joins in with her own baby noises.

- Experiment with different noises and see which she likes best.

- Dangle an object in front of her face, from about eight weeks you should see her follow it with her eyes.

- Read, sing and tell her stories – enjoy 'rhyme time' together or look for vocal singalong groups.

Introducing 'Bookbug'

Share books with your baby from the very first weeks – it's a great way to bond with her and a chance to have lots of hugs and cuddles together. Your health visitor/public health nurse will give you a Bookbug pack of free books when your baby is around 16 weeks old. The pack will give you some great ideas about good books to choose for your baby – as well as two free books to get you started!

Top tips

○ Talk to your baby about what you see on the page as well as reading the text – she'll have fun learning about all the different objects she can see.

○ Make noises to match the pictures – 'The duck says quack, the dog says woof'.

○ Match up what you see in the book to your baby's own experiences – 'Look, there's a picture of a dog – we saw a dog on our walk today'.

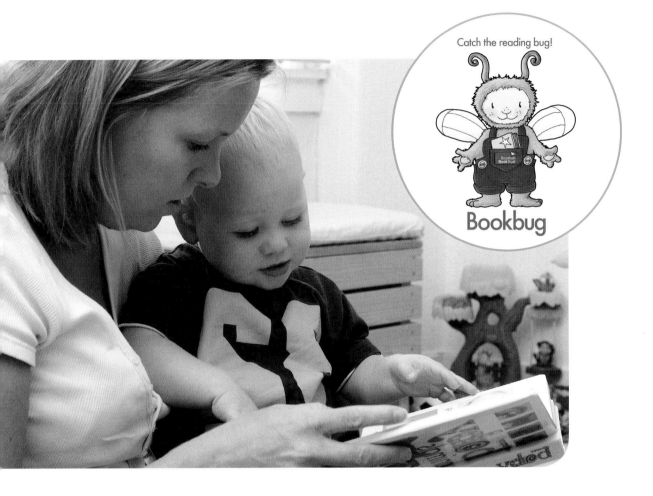

Catch the reading bug!

Bookbug

○ Don't worry about sounding silly – babies love to hear different voices, expressions and sounds.

○ Don't force your baby to look at books if she's not interested – try again later.

○ Leave her books out where she can reach them, so they become part of playtime – and don't worry if she chews them!

○ Keep your baby amused on a journey or in a queue by bringing a book to share.

Bookbug Sessions

Singing rhymes and songs to your baby is great fun, and good for her development. Hearing your voice is comforting and will help with her own speech and language development. Bookbug Sessions are a great way to join up with other parents and babies in your area. Ask at your local library for details, or log on to **www.scottishbooktrust.com**

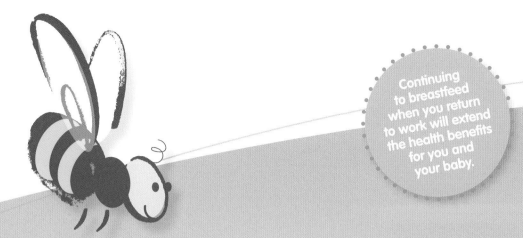

Continuing to breastfeed when you return to work will extend the health benefits for you and your baby.

What you can expect at
5–6 months

By the time your baby is five or six months old, you'll have a good understanding of her needs. You'll know the signs that mean she is tired, hungry, or wants attention. You may be in a routine by now which means you can tell when she will need feeding, or when she is due to have a sleep.

Many babies will be sleeping through the night by now, which is good news for their parents! Of course some nights she will still wake up, maybe because she is hungry, has a dirty nappy, or is feeling unwell.

When she cries, it's her way of telling you that something is not right.

Your baby will be smiling and laughing now when you play with her. And she'll show that she is annoyed or angry by squeaking or screaming, rather than by tearful crying.

She is becoming more sociable and will enjoy watching other children and show signs of wanting to join in. She is also thriving on your attention and is learning how to get more of it by waving or making a noise.

At six months your baby will be ready to start having 'solid' food, in addition to her regular breast or formula milk (see **Weaning your baby**, page 172).

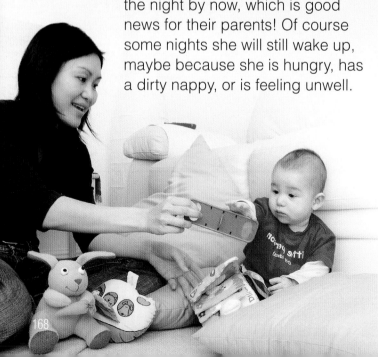

at **5–6** months your baby may be able to...

Remember not to leave your baby alone near a sharp or hard surface.

○ hold her arms out to be lifted

○ roll over from her front to her back and sometimes from her back to her front *(see page 187)*

○ sit up with support in the pram, or on the sofa with cushions around her (though don't leave her alone like this)

○ enjoy bouncing in a standing position on your lap

○ grasp small toys and objects that you put in front of her

○ drop something and let it fall – if she can't see it she'll forget it quickly, not realising she can look for it and find it again

○ know that if she shakes a rattle it makes a noise

○ use her mouth to explore everything, or put everything in her mouth

○ listen to more voices and start replying to you with sounds.

returning to work and continuing breastfeeding

Make sure that your employer can accommodate your choice to continue breastfeeding.

○ If your childcare is close to work this may mean arranging your work breaks to allow you to pop out to feed your baby.

○ If your childcare is not nearby, you may want to express milk at work. Your employer has a duty to provide a room or space where you can express milk, and a fridge where you can store it.

You can get more information from the NHS Health Scotland leaflet *Breastfeeding and returning to work* or by visiting **www.healthyworkinglives.com**.

Breastfeeding and returning to work

Off to a good start

healthier scotland   NHS

Remember!

○ You can provide expressed milk for your nursery or childminder to use. You may need to express milk at work, refrigerate it and then transport it in a sterilised container in a cool bag.

○ You can express milk during the day when you're at work, and breastfeed in the evening and at weekends when you and your baby are at home together – your body will soon adjust.

○ From six months, your baby can have expressed breast milk from a cup, so there's no need to introduce her to a bottle.

Childcare and babysitting

If you are returning to work full- or part-time, then you will have to consider childcare arrangements. You may be able to share the care with your partner or you may have a member of your family living close by who is prepared to help out. Alternatively, you may want to consider more formal arrangements such as a nursery or childminder.

Nurseries

Some mums choose to leave their baby in the care of a nursery when they return to work. Nurseries will typically have a few different rooms or areas so that your baby will be able to socialise with children her own age. It's a good idea to visit a few nurseries in your area to see which one you – and your baby – like best. But do remember that you may need to put your child's name down on a waiting list so it's worthwhile thinking ahead.

All good nurseries will be able to provide you with information about the daily activities and routines they will provide for your child, who her key carers will be, and how her needs will be met – feeding, naps, nappy changing and socialising. Make sure you are completely happy with what's on offer – and trust your own instincts too.

Childminders

Some mums choose to have their baby looked after by a childminder. Usually your baby will be looked after at the childminder's house – often in the company of other children – and often including the childminder's own. Make sure you are happy with the set-up at your childminder's house and with the number of other children being cared for.

With a childminder, your baby may have more of a 'home-from-home' routine which might include picking older children up from school, shopping and joining in with family activities.

It's important that you feel that the family's values match your own – trust your instincts, as well as your childminder's credentials.

Settling in

Going to nursery or a childminder is a big change for you and your baby, so arrange a settling in period before you go back to work – this allows you both to get used to the idea of being without each other for a few hours. You'll probably find this more of an emotional wrench than she does, so you could plan coffee with friends or shopping for new work clothes to enjoy that time to yourself!

Help with childcare

If you receive working tax credit, you may be eligible for financial help with the cost of registered childcare (registered through the Care Commission) through the childcare element of working tax credit. More information is available from the Inland Revenue, visit **www.inlandrevenue.gov.uk/taxcredits** or call **0845 300 3900**. Your local JobCentre Plus may also be able to help with the costs of childcare if you are looking for a job.

Childcare vouchers

If you need to find out about childcare vouchers, for the most up-to-date information look at **www.hmrc.gov.uk/childcare** which provides links to information and guidance about tax and National Insurance contributions (NICs) on employer-supported childcare (see page 64).

Registered childcare providers

The Care Commission has a list of registered childcare providers that you can access (**www.carecommission.com** or telephone **0845 60 30 890**). Your local Childcare Information Service (run by the local authority) can provide up-to-date advice on childcare and your options. There is a national website **www.scottishchildcare.gov.uk** which holds information on childcare and can direct you to your local Childcare Information Service. Your local JobCentre Plus can also advise on childcare options.

If you want to see a report on a particular nursery or childminder you can ask for the latest inspection reports or look at either the Care Commission or HMIE websites (**www.carecommission.com**) (**www.hmie.gov.uk**).

The type of childcare you choose will depend on your circumstances, the amount of money you have available and what sort of facilities there are locally.

Babysitting

You and your partner will want to enjoy some time alone together and so you may be looking for a babysitter.

In some areas, there are babysitting groups where mums get together and take it in turns to look after each other's children. Again, your health visitor/public health nurse will be able to tell you what's available locally. It's a good idea to spend some time with your new babysitter before you go out so that you and your child can get to know them. It's also helpful to point out any particular risks or hazards in your home.

Sometimes parents ask their older children to look after a younger brother or sister. If you're doing this, make sure they know how to get in touch with you and are aware of basics such as telephoning emergency services.

Make sure anyone you leave your child with knows where you are, when you'll be back and how to contact you. Also, leave a list of emergency numbers (for example, your GP) and ensure that the babysitter knows where the first aid box is and how to leave the house safely in case of fire.

babysitting and the law

The laws concerning who you can leave your baby with are not clear. Ultimately it's your responsibility to ensure your child is safe and well cared for. There is no provision in law specifying the age at which a child may either be left alone or may babysit. If you pay someone to babysit, they should be considered capable of doing so. If they are under 16, then you (as a parent) could be prosecuted if your child comes to any harm. If your babysitter is 16 or over, a court would generally assume that they were capable of looking after children. If they are babysitting, they have temporary care of your child and so also have a general responsibility to safeguard her health, development and welfare. But remember, this responsibility only applies if your babysitter is 16 or over.

Weaning your baby

Weaning is about introducing other food to your baby alongside her usual breast or formula milk. Until six months, breast or formula milk provides all the nourishment that babies need. At six months you can gradually introduce mashed foods (also known as 'solids'). However, you should continue to give your baby her regular formula milk feeds until she is at least a year old. You may continue to breastfeed your baby for as long as you wish.

Before six months, if you feel that your baby isn't satisfied with her usual milk feeds, give extra breast or formula milk rather than introduce solids too early.

Learning to eat

Just as your baby had to learn to feed from your breast or a bottle, so she needs to learn how to eat solid food. This is a gradual process which shouldn't be rushed. Be patient and allow your baby to develop her eating skills and tastes at her own pace. By her first birthday, your baby should be able to enjoy more or less the same food as the rest of the family. Developing a healthy approach to eating from the very start will stand her in good stead for the rest of her life.

When to start weaning

When your baby is approaching six months old (26 weeks) she may begin to show signs of being ready to eat solid food. For example, she can sit up, her eye and hand coordination allows her to reach out and grab things and she puts objects in her mouth and gnaws them. However, if your baby starts waking up in the night, when she used to sleep through, it's not necessarily a sign of hunger. Starting solids early will not help her to sleep longer or return to sleeping through the night.

Weaning at six months: the advantages

Medical evidence now suggests that waiting until six months carries significant health benefits.

- Weaning too early may increase the risk of asthma, eczema, digestive problems, allergies and obesity in later life.

- Chewing skills are more developed at six months so your baby will be able to have well-mashed food and move on to food with lumps and bumps.

- Chewing develops facial muscles which are later used for talking.

In addition, you'll enjoy some practical benefits if you wait until your baby is six months old – she'll have more control over her body, so feeding is easier when she can sit up in a high chair – and you don't have to sterilise all her feeding equipment.

Weaning early: the issues

If you choose to start giving your baby solid foods before six months (after talking to your health visitor or GP), don't give them any peanuts, nuts, seeds, milk, eggs, wheat, fish or shellfish, or any foods containing these products, until after six months of age. This is because these foods can sometimes trigger the development of a food allergy.

It is important that if you decide to wean before six months, that you discuss this with your health visitor first.

Babies under four months (17 weeks) should not be given solid food because they cannot digest it and you are replacing milk with less nutritious foods.

If you decide to wean earlier you will need to remember the following:

- All feeding equipment, including bowls and spoons will need to be sterilised.

- Younger babies need pureed foods and certain foods need to be avoided *(see page 174)*.

- All food will need to be pureed to a completely smooth, thin consistency until your baby is six months old. This may make it more difficult for her to progress on to mashed food, or food with lumps and bumps.

- If you wean at under six months, you'll need to feed your baby from a baby chair or while sitting on your lap, or sitting up supported by cushions on the floor.

How to start weaning

Like all the new experiences which you and your baby will enjoy together, it's best to start off slowly and work at a pace that suits both of you. Remember, it's not a race, so build up gradually from one 'solid' feed a day at first, to breakfast, lunch, tea and snacks by the time she is a year old. Some babies will take longer to do this than others.

Find a time that suits you

It's best not to give your baby solid food immediately before her regular milk feed – you don't want to fill her up and reduce her milk intake, as it's important that milk is the main part of her diet until she is a year old. Choose a time when she is awake and alert, but not expecting a milk feed. The middle of the day may be best.

Be safe and comfortable

At around six months, your baby will be able to support herself enough to sit in a high chair, safely strapped in. Don't leave her alone in her high chair, or leave her to feed herself – there's a very real danger that she could choke.

Spitting and refusing

When you first introduce solid food to your baby it is a completely new experience for her. As well as the unexpected taste and texture she has to learn to move the food around her mouth and swallow it. Many babies initially react by spitting their first mouthfuls of food straight back out again! This is quite normal and you should gently keep trying until she gets the hang of it. You might find that your baby refuses food at first. Again, this is fine. Leave it for another day and try again.

Your baby's appetite

Healthy babies know their own appetite and to begin with a couple of teaspoons of food may be enough. Never force your baby to eat if she doesn't want to – but do contact your health visitor/public health nurse if you're worried.

What to start with

A baby at six months can start off with mashed food – that is, food mashed with a fork to a soft consistency but with more texture than pureed food.

Suitable weaning foods

You don't have to buy any special foods for weaning your baby – lots of everyday foods are suitable. These include:

- baby rice mixed with your baby's usual milk

- cooked and mashed vegetables such as potato, sweet potato, carrot, parsnip or cauliflower

- peeled and mashed banana

- peeled, cooked and mashed fruit such as apple or pear.

Remember not to add any sugar or salt to your baby's food – salt can damage her kidneys.

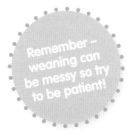
Remember – weaning can be messy so try to be patient!

What can my baby eat?

The table opposite shows foods which are unsuitable for your baby before six months, and indicates when they may be introduced. It is important that you do not introduce any of these foods before six months. This is because of possible allergic reaction. After six months you may gradually introduce these foods, one at a time, checking for any reaction. If you think your child is having an allergic reaction, you should seek urgent medical attention. Common symptoms of an allergic reaction include one or more of the following: coughing, dry itchy throat and tongue, itchy skin or rash, diarrhoea and/or vomiting, wheezing and shortness of breath, swelling of the lips and throat, runny or blocked nose, or sore red and itchy eyes.

Feeding and allergies

If your baby develops an obvious reaction just after eating a food for the first time, for example swelling or redness around the lips, you should report it to your health visitor/public health nurse or GP who will advise on whether any further investigations or precautions are necessary.

A severe and immediate allergic reaction such as anaphylaxis, that requires urgent medical care, is obvious. Medical staff will advise on how to check for possible causes and avoid repeat episodes. Some foods, such as honey, should be avoided altogether until your baby is over a year old.

Sometimes mothers remove foods from their baby's diet for various reasons. This is not always wise. It is always better to talk things over with your health visitor or GP before making any substantial changes to your baby's diet.

You may have heard about previous advice to avoid giving a child foods containing peanuts before three years of age, if there is a history of allergy in the child's immediate family (such as asthma, eczema, hayfever, food allergy or other types of allergy). This has now changed because the latest research has shown that there is no clear evidence to support this. If your child already has a known allergy, such as diagnosed eczema or a food allergy, then your child has a higher risk of developing a peanut allergy. In these cases, you should talk to your GP, health visitor, or medical allergy specialist before you give peanuts or foods containing peanuts to your child for the first time. Remember not to give whole peanuts, nuts or seeds to children under five because of the risk of choking.

For the most up-to-date advice on weaning your baby, ask your health visitor/public health nurse for a copy of the revised NHS Health Scotland leaflet, *Fun First Foods*. This booklet helps parents to introduce foods in a way that suits their child. It provides tips, advice, recipes and information on weaning.

Further information on food allergy, including peanut allergy, is provided on the Food Standards Agency website: www.eatwell.gov.uk/healthissues/foodintolerance/foodintolerancetypes/

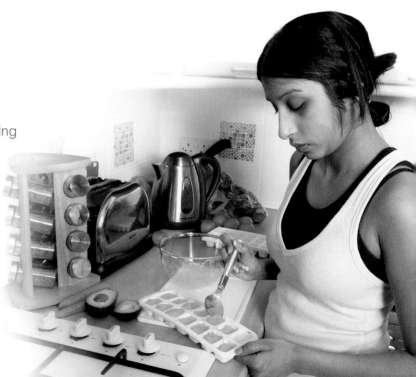

Food	Under 6 months	Over 6 months
Dairy products (cheese, plain fromage frais, custard, milk sauces and plain yoghurt)	No	Yes* cow's milk may be used in cooking but not to drink until at least a year old
Cereals that contain gluten, for example, wheat, rye, barley and oats, so avoid rusks, pasta, bread, flour, and breakfast cereals containing gluten, including porridge, until six months	No	Yes*
Follow-on formula, second-stage formula	No	No, not needed – continue breastfeeding or using formula
Citrus fruits (oranges, grapefruit) and juices	No	Yes* but juices diluted and kept to meal times
Soft berries (raspberries and strawberries)	No	Yes*
Fish and shellfish (for example, prawns)	No	Yes*
Eggs	No	Yes* and ensure they are always well cooked
Nut pastes, nut butter and ground nut oils	No	Yes*
Whole nuts and seeds	No	No, not until five years as risk of choking on nuts
Soya products (for example, tofu, soya yoghurt)	No	Yes*

*After six months you may gradually introduce this food, checking for any allergic reaction.

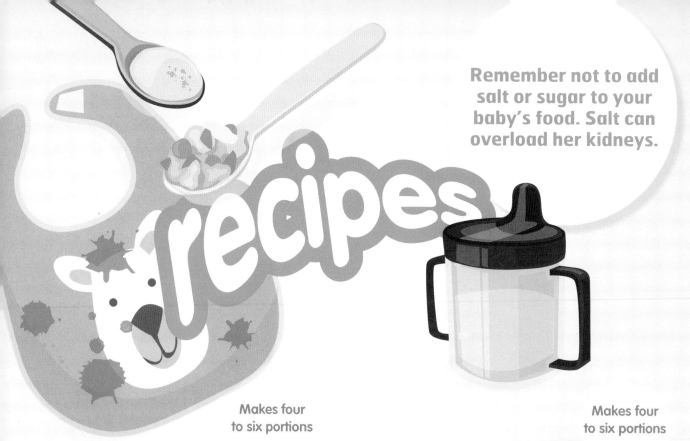

Remember not to add salt or sugar to your baby's food. Salt can overload her kidneys.

recipes

Makes four to six portions

Pear and peach mash

1 ripe pear, peeled and roughly chopped
205 g can of peach slices in fruit juice, drained – reserve juice

1. Roughly chop the peaches.
2. Place the pear and peaches in a small saucepan and add one tablespoon of the juice or water.
3. Simmer gently until the peaches are soft – about 15 minutes.
4. Drain off any liquid, reserving it.
5. Mash the fruit using the reserved liquid if needed.

Top tips from Daniella, mother of three, Glasgow

• **Cooking food – such as chicken and vegetables – in milk makes it easier to mash (but never add food to milk in bottles).**

• **Make several portions at once and freeze them in ice cube trays before storing them in food bags in the freezer.**

Makes four to six portions

Cauliflower, pea and potato mash

2 medium potatoes, peeled and quartered
2–3 florets cauliflower
100 g frozen peas
Milk, to taste

1. Cook the potatoes in boiling unsalted water for 15 minutes or until soft.
2. Cook the cauliflower by steaming or boiling in unsalted water for five minutes.
3. Add the peas to the cauliflower and bring the vegetables back to the boil. Cook for only a couple of minutes or until they are tender.
4. Drain the potatoes and mash with the milk. Do not add any salt.
5. Drain the cauliflower and peas, then mash.
6. Stir into the potato mash.

For variation, use broccoli instead of cauliflower, or replace peas with sweetcorn. For babies over six months you may add grated cheddar cheese.

Ready prepared foods

Baby foods can be expensive to use every day although it's possible to get healthy and interesting products. Read the label to check for added sugars, which make food very sweet, and for starch and water content – both bulk out the food but add little in the way of nutrition. Some babies who have a lot of pre-prepared 'baby food' take a while to get used to 'real' food with its varieties of tastes, textures and lumps.

Organic food

Some sources indicate that organic food may be better for us – and so for our babies. But it's not clear whether organic food is actually healthier, and it's certainly more expensive. Whatever you choose, it makes sense to buy the best and healthiest food you can afford.

Vegetarian diets

Babies do not need meat or fish to stay healthy, but you need to make sure she's getting enough protein and other nutrients from the rest of her diet. Make sure she gets a good variety of foods including pulses, eggs, milk, grains and cereals.

Vegan diets

A lot more care needs to be taken with a vegan diet, which cuts out animal products such as eggs and milk, although it is possible for your baby to develop healthily on such a diet. Ask your health visitor/public health nurse or GP to arrange for you to speak to a dietician if you are thinking of weaning your baby on to a vegan diet.

Feeding your growing baby

After six months you can start introducing your baby to foods she can pick up and eat by herself. Some babies seem to enjoy food better this way – they prefer picking things up and feeding themselves to taking food from a spoon. Getting your baby involved in feeding herself can also make weaning easier.

Here are a few suggestions for finger foods – all should be cut up into a shape and size your baby can hold easily to chew, gnaw or suck on:

- slices of bread, toast, chapatti or naan
- slices of eating apple or pear
- sticks of carrot or celery (part boiled)
- tiny sandwiches with grated cheese, cottage cheese or mashed banana
- fingers of cheese on toast or pizza
- cubes of cheese
- cooked pasta shapes
- cooked vegetables.

at a glance

✳ Solids don't replace milk – they are given in addition to it.

✳ Try to feed your baby on breast or formula milk alone until she is around six months old. If you feel your baby needs food before six months, discuss it with your health visitor/ public health nurse.

✳ Remember milk is still the most important part of her diet. She'll still need to be breastfed or have formula milk as the main milk drink each day until she's a year old. There are benefits both to your baby and to you if you continue breastfeeding for a year or more.

✳ From six months you can use full-fat cow's milk for cooking things like sauces and puddings but not for drinking until after her first birthday.

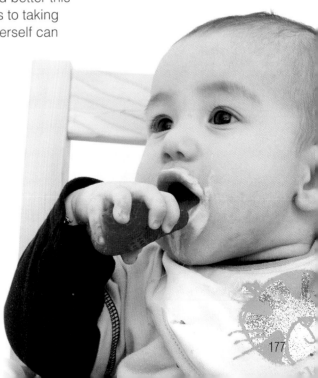

Teething

Teething normally starts between six and eight months but it can start earlier or later than this. It is not unusual for babies to be born with one or more teeth! It is also not unusual for babies not to have started teething by their first birthday. There are no hard and fast rules – all babies are different.

If your baby seems unusually quiet and unhappy, don't think it's just teething troubles. She may be ill. Contact your GP if she seems feverish.

Does teething cause pain?

Some babies sail through the process and are showing off their first teeth before you know it. For others it can be an uncomfortable time, causing distress to both you and your baby. For some babies, a day or two of restlessness can ease once a tooth has come through.

Some of the signs of teething you may see:

- dribbling more than usual
- flushed cheeks
- sore, red gums
- loss of appetite
- irritability and disturbed sleep
- chewing and biting on everything.

Easing teething

Here are some ways you can help to relieve your baby's discomfort:

- Cuddle her – hugs and cuddles will help comfort and reassure your baby if she is distressed.

- Rub her gums – lightly massaging your baby's gums with a clean finger will soothe her and help to alleviate the pain.

- Teething rings – babies like to chew and bite, so teething rings can help sometimes but make sure you watch your baby when she is biting on the ring.

- Sooth her sore chin – some babies may dribble excessively and give themselves a sore chin, neck and chest. Try to keep her chin as dry as possible and change any wet clothing. A simple barrier cream can help to keep her skin soft and smooth, and may ease chapped areas.

- Teething gels are not recommended.

Looking after your baby's teeth

From the moment her first tooth appears, you should brush your baby's teeth. Register her with a dentist as soon as possible and make sure she has regular check-ups with the dental team at least twice a year.

Brush your baby's teeth using a toothbrush with a small head and soft bristles. Add a smear of 1000 ppm fluoride toothpaste – fluoride helps to strengthen the teeth and prevent tooth decay. If you are not certain, ask your health visitor/public health nurse.

There are various ways to position your baby when you brush her teeth. You could try sitting her on a changing mat on the floor, on your lap or in a baby chair.

Toothbrushing should be introduced as a fun part of your baby's daily routine. You might find that a good time for toothbrushing is playtime or bathtime.

Make sure you brush her teeth last thing at night and at least once during the day. Always supervise toothbrushing and never leave a baby or small child alone with either a toothbrush or toothpaste.

To protect your baby's teeth, it's important to choose foods without added sugar. Sugar is the main cause of tooth decay, so don't give your baby sugary snacks, especially between meals. The safest drinks for your baby's teeth are milk and water.

Introduce a cup at six months and aim to have your baby no longer drinking from a feeding bottle by her first birthday. There's a risk that feeding from a bottle for too long can push your baby's new teeth out of alignment, so try and make sure that your baby has started drinking from a cup by the time she is about a year old. There is no risk to your baby's teeth from breastfeeding.

at a glance

❋ Start to brush your baby's teeth as soon as her first tooth appears.

❋ Use a soft toothbrush with a small head and a smear of 1000 parts per million (ppm) fluoride toothpaste.

❋ Protect your baby's teeth – don't encourage a sweet tooth.

❋ Register your baby with a dentist and arrange regular check-ups – at least twice a year.

❋ If you are unsure how to treat teething, please ask your health visitor/public health nurse or dentist.

Introducing 'Childsmile'

Childsmile is a dental programme designed to support you in giving your child's teeth the best possible start. Every child receives oral health packs, free-flowing drinking cups and daily supervised nursery toothbrushing. A variety of initiatives may be available in your area, including:

○ **access to Childsmile dental services for advice to support you in keeping your baby's teeth healthy**

○ **community oral health activities.**

For more information visit www.child-smile.org or see *Further help*, page 205.

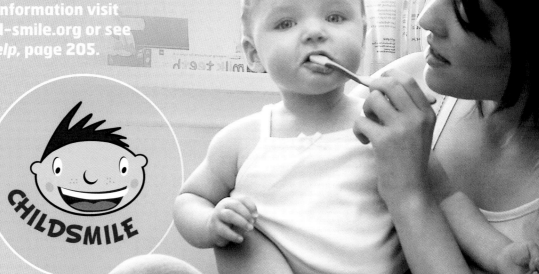

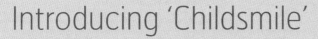

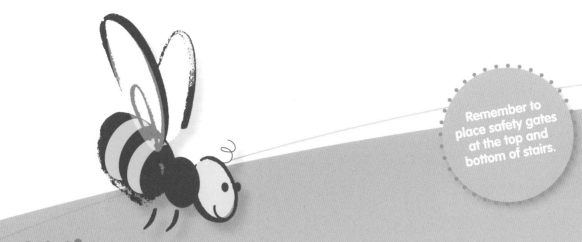

Remember to place safety gates at the top and bottom of stairs.

What you can expect at

7–8 months

At this stage you and your baby have really got to know each other. She's a real little person who can let you know what she likes and dislikes. You'll have clues about the type of child (and even adult!) she'll grow into – whether she'll be quiet and shy, or noisy and outgoing, whether she'll be easy-going or need constant entertainment and fun.

Like adults, she'll probably behave differently depending on what's going on and who she's with. Some babies get quite cranky at this point because they're beginning to realise what they can and can't do. She may really want to reach a toy on the other side of the room, for example, and get frustrated if she can't crawl yet. But that will come soon.

At around 7–8 months, some babies start to get shy with strangers – and upset if mum or dad leaves the room. This is very common. Your baby now feels very safe and secure with you, but less so with strangers, so she may turn away or bury her face in your shoulder because she feels a little bit anxious. For some babies, this shyness only lasts for a short time, for others it can be longer.

Similarly, if you leave the room, your baby will be anxious about whether you'll come back. She doesn't yet understand that you're still in the house – so call out to her to let her know you're around.

at **7–8** months your baby may be able to...

○ sit up without help for a few minutes

○ move across the floor by sliding, shuffling or rolling in some cases

○ hold and drink from a cup with a spout

○ look at where sounds are coming from quite accurately

○ react to familiar people around her and repeat an act if you praise her

○ babble and respond to you with noise

○ object loudly if you take a toy away from her – she will probably also protest if you leave her for too long

○ show extreme attachment to you and her regular carers – and not like anyone else!

○ roll over from back to tummy and from tummy to back

○ transfer objects from one hand to the other

○ support her whole weight on her legs when held upright

○ respond to her own name when you call it

○ explore objects with her hands and mouth

○ enjoy playing peek-a-boo

○ show an interest in mirror images.

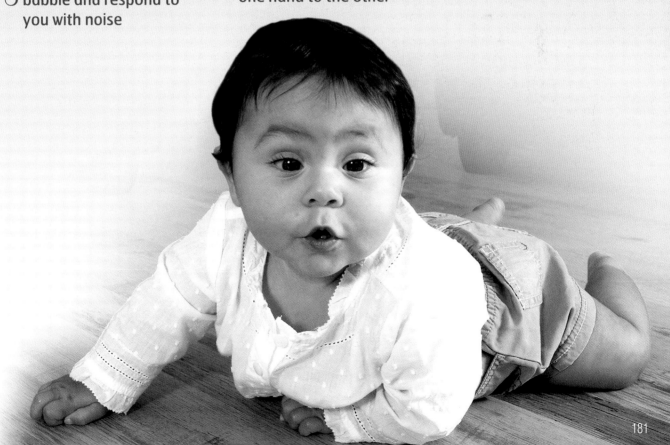

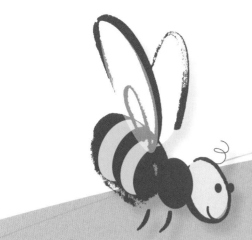

If your baby is eating less than usual, this is fine as long as she is happy and healthy and continues to grow. It's normal for your baby's appetite to change from day to day.

What you can expect at

9–10 months

By 10 months, most babies are either crawling or nearly there. Some can also 'cruise' around the furniture and pull themselves up to a standing position if furniture is the right height. Your baby may want to stick very close to your lap. She may still be a bit clingy at this stage if somewhere strange or with new people.

Your baby may also be getting more independent and able to make her feelings felt – for example, she may refuse to cooperate by stiffening her body as you try to dress her. She will also begin to use lots more gestures, including clapping and waving.

Experts believe introducing your baby to a wide range of foods early on can help her to enjoy a variety of tastes and textures – and make her less likely to be a picky eater later on in life! It might also help her to make healthier eating choices.

From now on, your baby will gradually start fitting in with your family eating patterns – eating breakfast, lunch, tea and maybe a couple of snacks in between.

at **9–10** months your baby may be able to...

○ turn and stretch to grasp a toy without toppling over

○ use her finger to point at small objects – babies also love poking their fingers into holes so make sure your electric sockets are covered

○ babble with recognisable sounds such as 'mama' and 'dada' and imitate noises that you make

○ understand some phrases such as 'no', 'bye-bye' and 'dinner', especially when they are part of a familiar routine, for example, she'll understand 'bath time' when she's in the bath

○ clap and wave – the beginnings of non-verbal communication

○ copy noises such as blowing raspberries and making kissing sounds

○ copy you to make the same thing happen, for example, show her how to ring a bell and she'll shake it to make the same noise

○ understand that things are still there even if she can't see them – she can watch while you hide a toy under a cloth and find it again by removing the cloth.

Playing with your baby at **9–10 months**

By now, babies are very interested in toys that have some sound and movement. They can use their fingers and hands to open little doors or to push things along. Show your baby what to do, and enjoyment and curiosity will make her copy you.

Have fun!

Check that play things are safe and can't be swallowed. Your baby will enjoy handing you items, and taking them from you as you hand them back. Playing with your baby is great fun – for her and for you – and it's a useful way to see how she is developing too.

Ideas for games

Babies enjoy finger games and hand games, such as 'Round and Round the Garden', and 'This Little Piggy'. They learn to look forward to the tickly bit at the end! Your baby may take your hand and make you do it again when you've stopped.

Clapping games help your baby's coordination skills. Help your baby to make music by singing and give her banging and rattling toys to join in with.

Play 'peep-bo' and 'boo', and watch the delight as your baby learns that, although you're hiding, you're still there.

Watch how your baby starts games. For example, babies learn that dropping a toy from a high chair means you pick it up… and, if they do it again, you pick it up again, and again, and again!

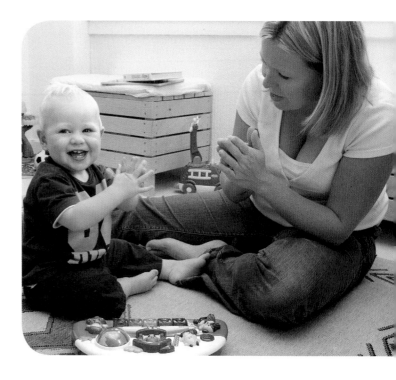

Your health visitor/public health nurse can help you with some ideas for games if you don't know any, or if you have forgotten them. It's an idea to switch off the television to reduce background noise when you're playing – and this is also true when you're reading to your child.

Ask your health visitor about play@home.

Building a 'busy box'

Put together a busy box for you to play with together. Talk about the things you're playing with, describe them and say what your baby's doing with them – 'Yes, you're touching that and it's all rough on that side, and this side's smooth...'

Here are some suggestions for your box – you can keep changing the items so there's always something new to study.

○ **Empty cotton reels**

○ **Small plastic bottles (throw tops away)**

○ **Scraps of different textured fabrics**

○ **Spoons**

○ **Doll's cup and saucer**

○ **Wooden bricks**

○ **Egg cartons**

○ **Ball**

○ **Crackly paper**

at a glance

✳ Put everyday items with different shapes and textures in a busy box.

✳ Enjoy playing finger and hand games to improve coordination.

✳ Sing and make music with your baby.

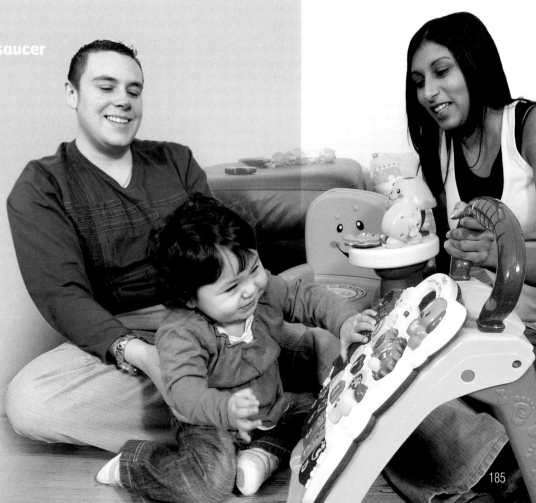

Safety and your growing baby

As your baby starts to grow and develop it's important to make sure that your home is safe and free from danger.

Use a door stop to prevent doors slamming on your child's fingers. Or tie a cloth across the front and back handles, which stops the door shutting completely.

Around the house

Here are some things to look out for, particularly when your baby starts to crawl, pull herself around the furniture, or walk.

○ Trailing flexes from electrical equipment – little hands can see them as a good thing to grab on to.

○ Modern electrical sockets have built-in safety shutters that come down when a plug is taken out. It is best to switch sockets off when they are not in use.

○ Hanging tablecloths.

○ Small objects, such as an older child's toys, left on the floor.

○ Hot drinks – don't let anyone drink them with a baby on their lap and don't leave them on low tables where they can be grabbed.

○ Blind cords – there's a danger they may trap your baby or strangle her.

Remember not to leave your baby alone with a family pet, however well they get on, and to keep stuff for your pets such as cat litter trays, food bowls and particularly water bowls, away from where your baby can get to them.

Action to take as your baby gets older:

• always place hot liquids, pans, tea and coffee pots well out of reach

• keep poisons such as medicine, tablets, cleaning materials and weedkillers out of reach and locked away

• keep garden tools out of reach and fill in or fence off garden ponds

• use a fire guard if you have a gas or open fire

• apply safety film or put safety glass on low-level glass surfaces, including doors and tables

• fit a guard over the controls of the TV, video and DVD

• put gates at the top and bottom of stairs.

For more advice and information, log on to the Child Accident Prevention Trust at **www.capt.org.uk**

When you're out and about

Remember that the law requires all children travelling in cars to use an appropriate child restraint for their size and weight *(see page 133)*. Visit **www.childcarseats.org.uk** for more information. And when you go for a bike ride, always wear cycle helmets.

Remember other people's houses and gardens won't necessarily be set up for baby safety so be watchful when you are out and about.

In the sun

Sun safety is even more important for your baby than it is for you. Babies under one year should be kept out of direct sunlight altogether and older babies and children should be protected.

The biggest risk of exposure to sunlight is sunburn. This is painful and can cause permanent damage or even skin cancer, which is becoming increasingly common. One episode of sunburn will double your baby's risk of developing skin cancer later in her life.

Keep her in the shade as much as possible and use a sunhat or sunshade on the pram or pushchair.

Use child sunscreen cream with a high protection factor (at least factor 25) and make sure your baby is covered up with at least a T-shirt and hat. Some manufacturers now sell bathing suits that cover up most of your child's body.

Other sensible precautions are staying indoors around midday in the summertime or when you're in a hot country and making sure your child gets plenty to drink in the heat.

Children and water

Children can drown in even a couple of inches of water. Never leave your baby alone in the bath or near water inside or outside the house, such as a garden pond or even a bucket. Also, it's an idea to set the temperature of your hot water tap lower than usual to make scalds less likely (see **Routine care – bathing**, page 134).

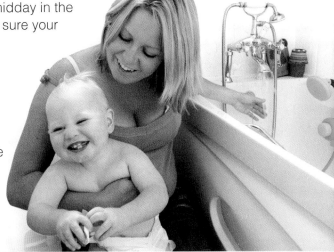

at a glance

❅ Make sure your house is safe and 'baby proof'.

❅ Always use high protection sunscreen and avoid hot midday sun.

❅ Use a car seat when travelling – and a cycle helmet if you go on a bike ride.

❅ Never leave your baby alone in or near water.

protect against bumps and falls

Never leave your baby (or later, your toddler) alone on a raised surface at any time. She may roll off and get hurt. Lots of mums and dads can be surprised when their baby learns to roll as it can happen suddenly. So it's sensible to be prepared.

Never leave your baby alone in bouncy seats or car seats or chairs placed on raised surfaces as there is a risk they can bounce or push themselves off. There are also risks to baby

walkers as babies can bump into things or even fall down stairs.

If you do use a baby walker, limit its use to short periods. Walkers won't help your baby to learn to walk, in fact using one too much may even slow her development slightly by delaying normal muscle control. A baby needs to roll, crawl, sit and play on the floor to reach her developmental milestones.

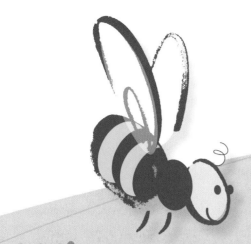

Baby's babble will begin to sound more like words and some babies will be using first words.

What you can expect at

11–12 months

Your baby has come on an amazing amount in just one year. As she approaches her first birthday, it's hard to believe it was only 12 months ago that she was a tiny helpless creature. Now she's grown, can do all sorts of things, can communicate with you, can get around – and very definitely has a mind of her own!

She'll be showing signs of wanting to make her own decisions – and won't always agree with you.

However, in lots of ways, babies do like to please and cooperate with you. You might find that your baby holds her arms out for her jacket, for example, or will wave bye-bye when asked to and may be able to point to familiar things.

You may want to think about how far you've come as parents in the past year and how well you've done. It's not been easy – but you've done a great job and had fun along the way!

Your health visitor/public health nurse may want to review your child's health and development at this stage if you have any concerns.

at **11–12** months your baby may be able to...

○ understand simple phrases such as 'Where is the cup?' and 'Do you want a drink?' and follow simple directions with familiar objects, for example, 'Bring me teddy'

○ recognise people she knows

○ show affection with kisses and cuddles

○ point to objects so that you can respond by commenting on them, for example 'Yes, that's a cup'

○ think it's fun to push, throw, and knock down everything in sight – giving toys to others or taking them away is also a new learning experience for her

○ use gestures like pointing and waving – this is also the stage where she'll understand more of what you are saying, including the word 'no'!

○ move around – some children learn to crawl during this stage, although others will develop more novel ways of getting around, such as creeping on their tummies, scooting on their bottoms, or rolling to wherever they want to go

○ walk by now – but don't worry if your baby isn't, it happens any time between eight and 20 months.

If your baby gets lots of new toys for her first birthday, put some of them away. This way, she's not overwhelmed by new things – and you've got some exciting toys up your sleeve for later!

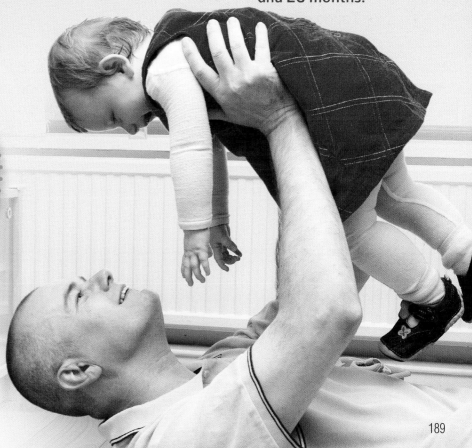

If your baby is ill

Babies who scream for a long time are worrying to parents, but babies who are really ill don't cry continuously and loudly. A baby who is really poorly is more likely to whimper and moan. Most babies (and parents!) will have off days.

Serious illnesses

Mild feverishness can bring on bouts of crying and usually it's not too much to worry about. Coughs and colds are common too – but it's the more serious (and rarely occurring) conditions that you need to be most aware of.

Telephone or see your GP if your baby:

- seems less bright and alert than usual or sleeps for an unusually long time

- is having bouts of vomiting for more than an hour

- has diarrhoea which doesn't clear up in a day

- has a rash which you can't explain as a heat rash or a result of clothes rubbing

- has dry nappies and does not seem to be passing as much urine as normal

- passes stools which are an unusual colour or texture for her or contain blood (green stools from time to time are not significant)

- seems feverish or uncomfortably hot

- has unexplained bruising or bleeding from the ears, mouth, nose or bottom, or blood in her stools or urine.

When in doubt, always seek help from your GP, health visitor/public health nurse. You can also call NHS 24, the 24-hour health service for Scotland on **08454 24 24 24**.

Seek medical help straight away if your baby:

- has a fit or convulsion – twitching or jerking with unfocused rolling eyes

- has breathing difficulties

- loses consciousness

- becomes blue around the lips or face

- has signs or symptoms of suspected meningitis or septicaemia *(see page 192)*

- passes blood or redcurrant jelly-like stools

- seems in obvious pain.

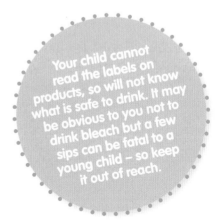

Your child cannot read the labels on products, so will not know what is safe to drink. It may be obvious to you not to drink bleach but a few sips can be fatal to a young child – so keep it out of reach.

> Jack had been off colour for a couple of days, but I didn't want to bother my GP in case he thought I was making a fuss about nothing. But he was so nice. Turns out Jack had an ear infection – and my GP said I'd done the right thing in bringing him in.
>
> *Paula, Glenrothes*

Medicine and your baby

Some over-the-counter remedies available at your pharmacist are especially for babies or small children. If in doubt, ask your pharmacist. Your GP won't prescribe medicine for your child if she doesn't need it. For example, antibiotics won't do anything to help a viral infection such as a cold or flu.

Safe storage of medicines

As a parent you will know only too well how young children like to put everything in their mouth. It is therefore very important that you keep all medicines safely stored out of reach of little hands. This also applies to the chemicals many of us leave under the kitchen sink – things such as bleach, disinfectants and polish.

It is also important to think about the other places in your home where you leave drugs or medicines – for example handbags, drawers or carrier bags of shopping left lying on the floor. Even everyday medications which you buy over-the-counter such as aspirin can be as dangerous as prescription drugs.

It is recommended that you store all tablets and other items that can be poisonous to a child in a sealed container in a secure place out of reach of curious fingers and mouths.

at a glance

❋ Mild illnesses such as coughs and colds are common.

❋ Life-threatening illnesses are very rare in babies and young children.

❋ Trust your instincts – if you're worried, seek help.

❋ There are times when your baby won't be well. As the person who knows your baby best, it's up to you to decide whether she's feeling ill and how seriously to take it.

Meningitis and septicaemia

Meningitis and septicaemia are very serious diseases that can affect anyone, of any age, very quickly. They are uncommon, but it is important to know the signs and symptoms and get medical help quickly.

What are meningitis and septicaemia?

Meningitis means swelling of the linings of the brain and spinal cord (meninges). Septicaemia is blood poisoning. These conditions can be caused by the same bacteria and viruses and can occur separately or together. Viral meningitis is more common than bacterial, but is less serious. If treated early enough, most children will survive.

Signs and symptoms of meningitis

The early signs and symptoms may be difficult to spot as they are similar to flu, but include:

- high-pitched moaning cry
- irritability when picked up
- bulging fontanelle (soft spot on baby's head)
- drowsy and non-responsive (difficult to wake)
- floppy/listless or stiff with jerky movements
- refusal to feed and vomiting
- fever, severe shivering and, or combined with, cold hands and feet
- 'staring' expression
- rapid breathing or difficulty breathing
- pin-prick rash or purple bruises on the body that do not fade under pressure (see glass test on opposite page)
- severe headache/dislike of bright lights.

Signs and symptoms of septicaemia

These will include:

- pale, blotchy, mottled skin
- irritability when picked up or handled due to joint/muscle pains
- bulging fontanelle (soft spot on baby's head)
- very drowsy and non-responsive (difficult to wake)
- floppy/listless or stiff with jerky movements
- refusal to feed and vomiting
- fever, severe shivering and cold hands/feet
- 'staring' expression
- rapid or unusual pattern of breathing
- red or purple bruise-like spots that do not fade under pressure (see glass test on opposite page).

Symptoms of meningitis or septicaemia can occur in any order. Not all babies develop all of the symptoms.

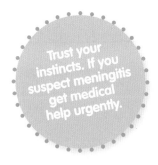

Trust your instincts. If you suspect meningitis get medical help urgently.

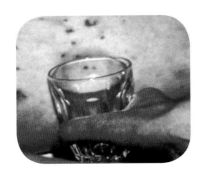

The 'glass test'

The rash, if present, starts as tiny red pinprick spots or marks and later changes to purple blotches, which can look like bruises or blood blisters. The rash can be anywhere. Press a clear drinking glass firmly against the rash so you can see if the rash fades and loses colour under pressure. If it doesn't change colour, contact your GP immediately. The spots and rash are more difficult to see on darker skin so check paler areas such as the palms of the hands, soles of the feet and the eye area. **Not everyone who gets meningitis will have this rash.**

What to do next

Remember that not all babies will develop the signs and symptoms listed on the facing page. If they develop some of them, especially the red or purple spots, get medical help urgently. If you can't get in touch with your GP or are still worried after getting advice, **trust your instincts** and take your baby to the emergency department of your nearest hospital. These conditions are dangerous and can develop very quickly. The earlier babies are treated, the better their chances of making a full recovery.

Prevention

Vaccines are available for meningitis and septicaemia but they don't protect against all forms.

PCV provides some protection against one of the commonest causes of meningitis, and also against other conditions such as severe ear infections (otitis media) and pneumonia caused by pneumococcal bacteria. This vaccine does not protect against all types of pneumococcal infection and does not protect against meningitis caused by other bacteria or viruses.

The Hib vaccine protects against Hib meningitis only and no other forms. The Men C vaccine protects against meningitis and septicaemia caused by meningococcal group C bacteria only.

More information

For further information call the NHS Helpline on **0800 22 44 88** or visit **www.nhs24.com/meningitis**

at a glance

✻ Meningitis is a very rare but serious illness.

✻ The majority of children will recover if diagnosed and treated early.

✻ Make sure you know the signs and symptoms; it could save your baby's life.

✻ Trust your instincts!

✻ If in doubt, seek medical help immediately.

What an incredible year!

Congratulations! You've now spent 12 months as a parent – and what an amazing amount you've learned. Practical things like feeding your baby, changing her nappy or bathing her – which seemed like huge challenges in the early days – will now be second nature. And the emotional challenges of parenthood – bonding with your baby, learning how to understand her needs, finding time for yourself and your partner – will have taught you a lot about yourself too. It's been an incredible year and you should be proud of how you've coped – and of what you've achieved.

It doesn't end here though. As your baby continues to grow and develop, you've a whole host of new experiences as a parent waiting for you. From toilet training to tantrums – and everything in between. As your baby becomes an independent little person and starts to walk, talk and express her feelings, you'll find our follow on publication **Ready Steady Toddler!** a great source of help and advice.

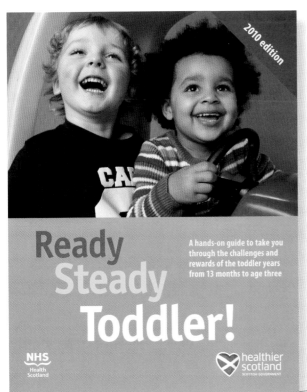

Ask your health visitor or public health nurse for a copy of **Ready Steady Toddler!** – like **Ready Steady Baby!** it was developed by health professionals and parents together, so is based on research and real experience. We hope you enjoy it, and find it useful on your journey as a parent.

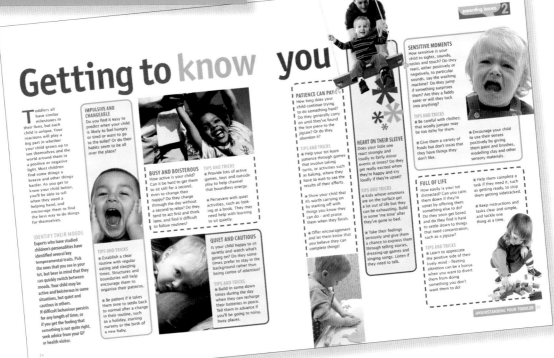

Further help: information and useful addresses

The following organisations may be able to put you in touch with local sources of help in your area. Those outside Scotland may have details of Scottish contacts. Call them for assistance and a friendly chat. Many of them provide leaflets on request. Where they exist, telephone helpline numbers have been included – you may wish to contact them for advice, counselling or for general information.

A very useful service which provides information about where to find help is available through your local health education/promotion unit which is listed under 'Health' in your phone book and/or the **NHS Helpline Freephone: 0800 22 44 88** (all calls are free of charge 8 am–10 pm, seven days). Your public library is also an invaluable source of information. For further information about any health-related issues, please contact:

NHS Health Scotland Library
The Priory
Canaan Lane
Edinburgh EH10 4SG
Tel: 0131 536 5581
Textphone: 0131 536 5593
email: nhs.healthscotland-library@nhs.net
www.healthscotland.com/library

ABUSE

Children 1st

83 Whitehouse Loan
Edinburgh EH9 1AT
Tel: 0131 446 2300
Email: info@children1st.org.uk
www.children1st.org.uk

Offers practical help to families
with children at risk.

Domestic Violence

National Helpline (24hr):
0808 200 0247

ParentLine Scotland

0808 800 2222

Confidential and anonymous
telephone helpline run by
volunteers for parents/carers.

Scottish Women's Aid

2nd Floor, 132 Rose Street
Edinburgh EH2 3JD
Tel: 0131 226 6606
Email: info@scottishwomensaid.org.uk
www.scottishwomensaid.org.uk

Advice, support and refuge for
women who have been abused
mentally, physically or sexually
(by their partner or ex-partner),
and their children.

ACCIDENT PREVENTION AND SAFETY

British Red Cross Society (Scottish Region)

4 Nasmyth Place
Hillington
Glasgow G52 4PR
Tel: 0141 891 4000
www.redcross.org.uk

Provides a range of caring and
first-aid services and courses.

Child Accident Prevention Trust (CAPT)

4th Floor, Cloister Court
22–26 Farringdon Lane
London EC1R 3AJ
Tel: 020 7608 3828
Email: safe@capt.org.uk
www.capt.org.uk

Offers help and advice to
parents on the prevention
of childhood accidents.

Home Safety Scotland

www.homesafetyscotland.org.uk

The Scottish organisation working
to reduce deaths and injuries in
the home.

Iain Goodwill Trust

Viewfield
Pettyvaich
Kiltarlity
Beauly IV4 7HU
Tel: 01463 741 854
Email: info@ians-trust.org
www.iains-trust.org

Campaigns on car safety issues to
prevent accidents.

The Royal Society for the Prevention of Accidents (RoSPA)

Livingstone House
43 Discovery Terrace
Heriot-Watt University Research Park
Edinburgh EH14 4AP
Tel: 0131 449 9378
www.rospa.com

Information and advice on
the prevention of accidents
of all kinds.

St Andrew's Ambulance Association

St Andrew's House
48 Milton Street
Glasgow G4 0HR
Tel: 0141 332 4031
Email: firstaid@staaa.org.uk
www.firstaid.org.uk

Provides training in first
aid and related subjects.

Scottish Road Safety Campaign

Heriot-Watt Research Park (North)
Riccarton
Currie
Edinburgh EH14 4AP
Tel: 0131 472 9200
Email: enquiries@roadsafety.org.uk
www.roadsafetyscotland.org.uk

A campaign to develop and
coordinate Scotland-wide
road safety initiatives.

ADOPTION

Scottish Adoption Association

161 Constitution Street
Edinburgh EH6 7AD
Tel: 0131 553 5060
Email: info@scottishadoption.org
www.scottishadoption.org

Offers a comprehensive adoption
service including advice and
counselling to anyone affected
by adoption.

ALCOHOL, DRUGS AND SMOKING

Alcohol Focus Scotland

2nd Floor, 166 Buchanan Street
Glasgow G1 2LW
Tel: 0141 572 6700
Email: enquiries@alcohol-focus-scotland.org.uk
www.alcohol-focus-scotland.org.uk

Provides free, confidential
counselling services for people
affected by alcohol problems.
Promotes safer, healthier drinking
styles, but is not anti-alcohol.

Alcoholics Anonymous (AA)

Baltic Chambers
50 Wellington Street
Glasgow G2 6HJ
Tel: 0141 226 2214
Helpline: 0845 769 7555
www.alcoholics-anonymous.org.uk

Network of self-help groups where
members encourage each other
to stop drinking and to stay off drink.
Look in the phone book for details
of your local group.

Can stop smoking.com

www.canstopsmoking.com

Advice and support for stopping smoking, including local details for stop smoking services.

FRANK (National drugs helpline)

0800 77 66 00
Email: frank@talktofrank.com
www.talktofrank.com

Free 24-hour confidential drug information, advice and counselling service.

Scottish Drugs Forum

91 Mitchell Street
Glasgow G1 3LN
Tel: 0141 221 1175
Email: enquiries@sdf.org.uk
www.sdf.org.uk

Offers information on local treatment and services for drug users, family and friends.

Smokeline

0800 84 84 84

Scottish national helpline for smokers who need advice or help in stopping, or for their friends who are encouraging them to stop. Provides details of local services.

BEHAVIOURAL DIFFICULTIES

Hyperactive Children's Support Group

71 Whyke Lane
Chichester
West Sussex PO19 7PD
Tel: 01243 539966
Email: hacsg@hacsg.org.uk
www.hacsg.org.uk

Provides information and ideas to parents and professionals about nutritional/dietary therapies for hyperactive and allergic children.

BREASTFEEDING

Association of Breastfeeding Mothers (ABM)

PO Box 207
Bridgwater
Somerset TA6 7YT
Helpline: 08444 122 949
Email: counselling@abm.me.uk
www.abm.me.uk

Gives support and information to all women wishing to breastfeed, and offers counselling around the UK.

The Breastfeeding Network

PO Box 11126
Paisley PA2 8YB
Supportline: 0300 100 0210
www.breastfeedingnetwork.org.uk

Offers independent information and support about breastfeeding.

La Leche League (Great Britain)

PO Box 29
West Bridgford
Nottingham NG2 7NP
Helpline: 0845 120 2918
Email: enquiries@laleche.org.uk
www.laleche.org.uk

Help and information for women wanting to breastfeed their babies and personal counselling to mothers having problems in breastfeeding.

National Childbirth Trust (NCT)

Alexandra House
Oldham Terrace
Acton
London W3 6NH
Breastfeeding: 0870 444 8708
Email: enquiries@nct.org.uk
www.nct.org.uk

Help and information for women wanting to breastfeed their babies.

UNICEF UK Baby Friendly Initiative

Africa House
64–78 Kingsway
London
WC2B 6NB
Tel: 020 7312 7652
Email: bfi@unicef.org.uk
www.babyfriendly.org.uk

Works with health services to improve practice so that parents are enabled and supported to make informed choices about how they feed and care for their babies.

CHILDCARE

National Association of Toy and Leisure Libraries

First Floor
Gilmerton Community Centre
4 Drum Street
Edinburgh EH17 8QG
Tel: 0131 664 2746
Email: natll.scotland@playmatters.co.uk
www.natll.org.uk

Toy libraries loan good quality, carefully chosen toys to all families with babies and young children, including those with special needs.

Scottish Childminding Association

7 Melville Terrace
Stirling FK8 2ND
Helpline: 01786 449063
(Mon/Fri 10.00 – 16.00)
Email: information@childminding.org
www.childminding.org

An association committed to meeting the needs of registered childminders and actively promoting childminding as a quality childcare choice.

Scottish Preschool Play Association

21 Granville Street
Glasgow G3 7EE
Tel: 0141 221 4148
Email: info@sppa.org.uk
www.sppa.org.uk

An organisation for playgroups, mother-and-toddler groups and under-fives groups in Scotland.

Scottish Out of School Care Network

Level 2, 100 Wellington Street
Glasgow G2 6DH
Tel: 0141 564 1284
Email: info@soscn.org
www.soscn.org

A Scottish charity supporting school-aged play, care and learning, which promotes, supports and develops good quality sustainable out-of-school care.

Care Commission

Compass House
11 Riverside Drive
Dundee DD1 4NY
Tel: 01382 207100
Helpline: 0845 6030890
www.carecommission.com

A national organisation which regulates and inspects Scottish care services including childcare services.

DISABILITY AND ILLNESS (GENERAL SUPPORT)

Action for Sick Children (Scotland)

22 Laurie Street
Edinburgh EH6 5AB
Tel: 0131 553 6553
Freephone: 0800 0744519
www.actionforsickchildren.org

Supports sick children and their families. Offers information about going to hospital, designed for children and for parents. Hospital playboxes available for borrowing by playgroups.

Contact a Family Scotland

Craigmillar Social Enterprise & Art Centre (SPACE)
11/9 Harewood Road
Edinburgh EH16 4NT
Tel: 0131 659 2930
Helpline: 0808 808 3555
Email: scotland@cafamily.org.uk
www.cafamily.org.uk

Encourages mutual support between families caring for children with any type of disability or special need.

ENABLE

2nd Floor, 146 Argyle Street
Glasgow G2 8BL
Tel: 0141 226 4541
Email: enable@enable.org.uk
www.enable.org.uk

Promotes the rights and needs of people with learning disabilities and their families. Can offer information, advice and practical help.

Family Fund

Unit 4, Alpha Court
Monks Cross Drive
Huntington Drive
York YO32 9WN
Tel: 0845 130 4542
Email: info@familyfund.org.uk
www.familyfund.org.uk

Textphone users can call: 01904 658085.

A government-funded trust whose purpose is to ease the stress on families who care for severely disabled children under 16 by providing grants and information related to the care of the child.

Genetic Interest Group (GIG)

Unit 4D, Leroy House
436 Essex Road
London N1 3QP
Tel: 020 7704 3141
Email: mail@gig.org.uk
www.gig.org.uk

Information service for people with, or at risk of, genetic conditions.

Sleep Scotland

8 Hope Park Square
Edinburgh EH8 9NW
Tel: 0131 651 1392
Email: enquiries@sleepscotland.org
www.sleepscotland.org

Provides support to families with children with special needs and severe sleep problems.

DISABILITY AND ILLNESS (SPECIALISED SUPPORT)

Advice Service Capability Scotland (ASCS)

11 Ellersly Road
Edinburgh EH12 6HY
Tel: 0131 313 5510
Email: ascs@capability-scotland.org.uk
www.capability-scotland.org.uk

Offers advice, support and information to parents of children with cerebral palsy.

AFASIC Unlocking Speech and Language

1st Floor, 20 Bowling Green Lane
London EC1R 0BD
Helpline: 0845 3 55 55 77
Tel (admin): 020 7490 9410
Email: info@afasic.org.uk
www.afasic.org.uk

Provides advice and information on speech and language difficulties among children.

Anaphylaxis Campaign

PO Box 275
Farnborough GU14 6SX
Tel: 01252 546100
Helpline: 01252 542029
Email: info@anaphylaxis.org.uk
www.anaphylaxis.org.uk

Campaigns to help anyone who suffers from a potentially fatal allergy. Provides help to sufferers and aims to raise awareness within government, industry and the general public.

Scottish Association for Children with Heart Disorders

104 Comiston Road
Edinburgh EH10 5QL
Email: secretary@youngheart.info
www.youngheart.info

Provides support to children and young adults with heart disorders, and their families.

Asthma UK Scotland

4 Queen Street
Edinburgh EH2 1JE
Tel: 0131 226 2544
Helpline: 0845 701 0203
Email: scotland@asthma.org.uk
www.asthma.org.uk

Information and support for people with asthma and their families.

Child Growth Foundation

2 Mayfield Avenue
Chiswick
London W4 1PW
Tel: 020 8995 0257
Email: info@childgrowthfoundation.org
www.childgrowthfoundation.org

Support group for parents of children with growth disorders, and parents concerned about their child's growth.

Children Living with Inherited Metabolic Diseases (CLIMB)

Climb Building
176 Nantwich Road
Crewe CW2 6BG
Tel: 0800 652 3181
Email: Info.svcs@climb.org.uk
www.climb.org.uk

Makes grants and allowances available for the purposes of medical treatment and care of children with metabolic diseases. Puts parents in contact with others in similar circumstances.

Cleft Lip and Palate Association (CLAPA)

CLAPA Head Office
1st Floor, Green Man Tower
332b Goswell Road
London EC1V 7LQ
Tel: 020 7833 4883
Email: info@clapa.com
www.clapa.com

Offers support to parents of children with cleft lip and/or palate. Offers a specialist service to those seeking help in feeding babies with clefts.

The Coeliac Society

Suites A-D
Octagon Court
High Wycombe
Bucks HP11 2HS
Helpline: 0870 444 8804
www.coeliac.co.uk

Advice and information for those with a coeliac condition or dermatitis herpetiformis.

Craighalbert Centre

The Scottish Centre for Children with Motor Impairments
1 Craighalbert Way
Cumbernauld G68 0LS
Tel: 01236 456100
Email: sccmi@craighalbert.org.uk
www.craighalbert.org.uk

A Scottish national centre that offers a system of 'conductive education' which aims to teach the cerebral palsied child all aspects of daily life, develop learning ability and prepare the child for school.

Cystic Fibrosis (CF) Trust

11 London Road
Bromley
Kent BR1 1BY
Tel: 020 8464 7211
Email: enquiries@cftrust.org.uk
www.cftrust.org.uk

Funds medical and scientific research aimed at understanding, treating and curing cystic fibrosis. Aims to ensure that people with CF receive the best care and support in all aspects of their lives.

The Butterfly Trust

Swanston Steading
109/3B Swanston Road
Edinburgh EH10 7DS
Tel: 0131 445 5590
Email: info@butterflytrust.org.uk
www.butterflytrust.org.uk

A charity which offers advice, practical help and advocacy to people with cystic fibrosis and their families.

Diabetes UK Scotland

Savoy House
140 Sauchiehall Street
Glasgow G2 3DH
Careline: 0845 120 2960
Tel: 0141 332 2700
Email: scotland@diabetes.org.uk
www.diabetes.org.uk/scotland

Provides practical help and information on living with diabetes.

Down's Syndrome Scotland

158–160 Balgreen Road
Edinburgh EH11 3AU
Tel: 0131 313 4225
Email: info@dsscotland.org.uk
www.dsscotland.org.uk

Information, advice, counselling and support for parents of children with Down's syndrome.

National Eczema Society

Hill House
Highgate Hill
London N19 5NA
Helpline: 0800 089 1122
Tel: 020 7281 3553
Email: helpline@eczema.org
www.eczema.org

Information, advice and support for people with eczema and their families.

Epilepsy Scotland

Head Office
48 Govan Road
Glasgow G51 1JL
Tel: 0141 427 4911
Helpline: 0808 800 2200
Email: enquiries@epilepsyscotland.org.uk
www.epilepsyscotland.org.uk

A charitable organisation working for people with epilepsy, their families, carers and the professionals looking after them.

Group B Strep Support

PO Box 203
Haywards Heath
West Sussex RH16 1GF
Tel: 01444 416176
Email: info@gbss.org.uk
www.gbss.org.uk

Provides information for pregnant women, pregnant women who carry the bacteria, parents of infected children and healthcare professionals.

The Haemophilia Society

First Floor, Petersham House
57a Hatton Garden
London EC1N 8JG
Tel: 020 7381 1020
Helpline: 0800 018 6068
Email: info@haemophilia.org.uk
www.haemophilia.org.uk

Represents the needs and interests of people with, or affected by, haemophilia.

Jennifer Trust for Spinal Muscular Atrophy (SMA)

Elta House
Birmingham Road
Stratford Upon Avon CV37 0AQ
Freephone Helpline: 0800 975 3100
Tel: 01789 267 520
Email: jennifer@jtsma.org.uk
www.jtsma.org.uk

For those affected by any form of SMA. Can link families and help to provide equipment.

MENCAP, the Learning Disability Charity

Mencap
123 Golden Lane
London EC1Y 0RT
Tel: 020 7454 0454
Email: information@mencap.org
www.mencap.org.uk

Works with children and adults with a learning disability and their families and carers to improve their lives and opportunities.

Meningitis Association of Scotland

9 Edwin Street
Glasgow G51 1ND
Tel: 0141 427 6698
Email: info@menscot.org
www.meningitis-scotland.org

Free information and support to those suffering from meningitis or who are disabled as a result.

Meningitis Research Foundation

28 Alva Street
Edinburgh EH2 4PY
Tel: 0131 510 2345
Helpline: 080 8800 3344/
0131 510 2345
Email: info@scotland.meningitis.org.uk
www.meningitis.org.uk

Offers counselling for parents whose children have died from meningitis and gives support to people with loved ones in hospital or at home (see Meningitis Trust, below).

Meningitis Trust

Centrum Offices Ltd
38 Queen Street
Glasgow G1 3DX
Helpline: 0800 028 1828
Email: info@meningitis-trust.org
www.meningitis-trust.org

Free information and support to those suffering from meningitis or who are disabled as a result.

Muscular Dystrophy Campaign

61 Southwark Street
London SE1 0HL
Information and Support Line: 0800 652 6352 (Freephone)
Tel: 020 7803 4800
Email: info@muscular-dystrophy.org
www.muscular-dystrophy.org

Offers practical help and emotional support to sufferers and their families, runs an information and education service for the medical professions, social services and the public.

National Autistic Society Scotland

Central Chambers
1st Floor, 109 Hope Street
Glasgow G2 6LL
Tel: 0141 221 8090
Email: scotland@nas.org.uk
www.nas.org.uk

A parent support group which runs an advisory and information service.

National Deaf Children's Society Scotland

187–189 Central Chambers
93 Hope Street
Glasgow G2 6LD
Tel: 0141 248 4457
Minicom: 0141 222 4476
Helpline: 0808 800 8880 (voice or text)
Email: ndcs.scotland@ndcs.org.uk
www.ndcs.org.uk

Offers information and advice on all issues relating to childhood deafness. Offers the expertise of specialist advisors in the fields of education, health, benefits and technology.

National Society for Phenylketonuria (NSPKU)

PO Box 26642
London N14 4ZF
Helpline: 0208 364 3010
Recorded Info: 0207 099 7431
Email: info@nspku.org
Text: 07983 688664
www.nspku.org

A self-help organisation offering information and support to families affected by the disorder.

Reach (Association for Children with Hand or Arm Deficiency)

PO Box 54
Helston
Cornwall TR13 8WD
Tel: 0845 1306 225
Email: reach@reach.org.uk
www.reach.org.uk

Aims to promote the relief of children with upper limb deficiencies by encouraging mutual aid and support between their families.

RNIB Scotland

Dunedin House
25 Ravelston Terrace
Edinburgh EH4 3TP
Tel: 0131 311 8500
Email: rnibscotland@rnib.org.uk
www.rnib.org.uk

Information, services and advice for blind people. Look Scotland (0131 313 5711) provides information to parents on services relevant to children with visual impairment.

Scope

6 Market Road
London N7 9PW
Scope Response: 0808 800 3333
Email: response@scope.org.uk
www.scope.org.uk

Provides a range of services for people with cerebral palsy and their families/carers.

Scottish Society for Autism

Hilton House
Alloa Business Park
Whins Road
Alloa FK10 3SA
Tel: 01259 720044
Email: info@autism-in-scotland.org.uk
www.autism-in-scotland.org.uk

Provides a range of services in care, support and education for people with autism, their families and carers.

Scottish Spina Bifida Association

The Dan Young Building
6 Craighalbert Way
Cumbernauld G68 0LS
Tel: 01236 794 500
Helpline: 08459 111112
Email: mail@ssba.org.uk
www.ssba.org.uk

Information, advice, counselling, support and financial help for parents.

SENSE Scotland (National Deaf–Blind and Rubella Association)

43 Middlesex Street
Kinning Park
Glasgow G41 1EE
Tel: 0141 429 0294
Textphone: 0141 418 7170
Email: info@sensescotland.org.uk
www.sensescotland.org.uk

Information, advice and support for families of deaf–blind and rubella-handicapped children.

Sickle Cell Society

54 Station Road
London NW10 4UA
Tel: 020 8961 7795
Email: info@sicklecellsociety.org
www.sicklecellsociety.org

Information, advice and counselling on sickle cell disease and traits.

Society for Mucopolysaccharide Diseases (MPS)

MPS House
Repton Place
White Lion Road
Amersham
Buckinghamshire HP7 9LP
Tel: 0845 389 9901
Email: mps@mpssociety.co.uk
www.mpssociety.co.uk

Acts as a parent support group; brings about more public awareness of MPS diseases; raises funds for research.

UK Thalassaemia Society

19 The Broadway
Southgate Circus
London N14 6PH
Tel: 020 8882 0011
Email: office@ukts.org
www.ukts.org

Education, information, research and counselling offered to sufferers and carriers.

FAMILY PLANNING

Caledonia Youth

5 Castle Terrace
Edinburgh EH1 2DP
Tel: 0131 229 3596
Email: edinburgh@caledoniayouth.org
www.caledoniayouth.org

Confidential support in both educational and clinical environments, enabling all young people in Scotland to make informed, responsible choices about their personal and sexual relationships.

Family Planning Association Scotland

Unit 10, Firhill Business Centre
76 Firhill Road
Glasgow G20 7BA
Helpline: 0141 948 1179
www.fpa.org.uk

Aims to promote sexual, emotional and reproductive health, together with planned parenthood, by providing information, publicity, education and training.

GENERAL SUPPORT

AskBaby.com

All you need to know about getting pregnant, coming off the Pill and fertility problems.

Caesarean Support Network

55 Cooil Drive
Douglas
Isle of Man IM2 2HF
Tel: 01624 661269 (evenings only)

Provides support and advice on all matters relating to Caesarean delivery, whether recent or in the past.

DirectGovUK

www.direct.gov.uk

Advice on preparing for pregnancy and conceiving.

Family Mediation Scotland

Tel: 0845 119 2020
Email: info@familymediationscotland.org.uk
www.familymediationscotland.org.uk

Relate Scotland

18 York Place
Edinburgh EH1 3EP
Tel: 0845 119 6088
Email: enquiries@relatescotland.org.uk
www.relatescotland.org.uk

Offers advice, relationship counselling, sex therapy, consultations and support face-to-face, by phone and through their website.

Scottish Marriage Care

72 Waterloo Street
Glasgow G2 7DA
Tel. 0141 222 2166
www.scottishmarriagecare.org

Institute for Complementary Medicine

PO Box 194
London SE16 1QZ
Tel: 020 7231 5855
Email: info@i-c-m.co.uk
www.i-c-m.org.uk

Charity providing information on complementary medicine and referrals to qualified practitioners or helpful organisations.

Life

Life House
Newbold Terrace
Leamington Spa CV32 4EA
Helpline: 0800 915 4600
Email: info@lifecharity.org.uk
www.lifecharity.org.uk

Offers free, confidential information, counselling and support for women contemplating abortion, suffering after pregnancy loss or struggling to cope after abortion.

NHS 24

Tel: 08454 24 24 24
www.nhs24.com

Information on pregnancy, childbirth and infections during pregnancy.

NHS UK

www.nhs.uk

Pregnancy and childbirth advice.

The Baby Website

www.thebabywebsite.com

Provides information on a range of topics from breastfeeding to baby names.

The Infertility Network

Charter House
43 St Leonards Road
Bexhill-on-Sea
East Sussex TN40 1JA
Tel: 0800 008 7464
Email: admin@infertilitynetwork.uk.com
www.infertilitynetworkuk.com

Helps couples coping with problems of infertility and childlessness.

Scotland Patients' Association

PO BOX 2817
Glasgow G61 9AY
Tel: 0141 942 0376, between 9.30 am–4.30 pm, Monday to Friday
www.scotlandpatients.com

Provides patients with an opportunity to raise concerns about healthcare.

Shelter Scotland

4th Floor, Scotiabank House
6 South Charlotte Street
Edinburgh EH2 4AW
Helpline: 0808 800 4444
Email: edinburgh_shac@shelter.org.uk
www.shelter.org.uk

Works to relieve poverty and distress among homeless people and campaigns for provision of housing to meet need; runs regional housing aid offices and charity shops.

Stepfamily Scotland

Gillis Centre
113 Whitehouse Loan
Edinburgh EH9 1BB
Helpline: 0845 122 8655
Email: info@stepfamilyscotland.org.uk
www.stepfamilyscotland.org.uk

If you are in a stepfamily already, or about to become part of one, Stepfamily Scotland can provide helpful advice and support.

Men's Advice Line and Enquiries (MALE)

1st Floor, Downstream Building
1 London Bridge
London SE1 9BG
Helpline: 0808 801 0327
Email: info@mensadviceline.org.uk
www.mensadviceline.org.uk

Open 10 am–1 pm, 2 pm–5 pm on Mondays, Tuesdays and Wednesdays.

Provides information, support and advice for men experiencing domestic abuse.

HIV AND AIDS

National Aids Trust

New City Cloisters
196 Old Street
London EC1V 9FR
Tel: 020 7814 6767
Email: info@nat.org.uk
www.nat.org.uk

Aims to promote a wider understanding of HIV and AIDS; to develop and support efforts to prevent the spread of HIV; and to improve the quality of life of people affected by HIV and AIDS.

Positive Voice

37–39 Montrose Terrace
Edinburgh EH7 5DJ
Tel: 0131 652 0754
Email: enquiries@positive-voice.org.uk
www.positive-voice.org.uk

Offers support, advice and counselling to those who are affected by HIV, AIDS or Hepatitis.

Positively Women

347–349 City Road
London EC1V 1LR
Helpline: 020 7713 0444
Email: info@positivelywomen.org.uk
www.positivelywomen.org.uk

Support agency for women living
with HIV/AIDS and their families.

Waverley Care Solas

2–4 Abbeymount
Edinburgh EH8 8EJ
Tel: 0131 661 0982
Email: info@waverleycare.org

Waverley Care Head Office

Old Coates House
32 Manor Place
Edinburgh EH3 7EB
Tel: 0131 226 2206
Email: info@waverleycare.org
www.waverleycare.org

Supporting people in Scotland
living with HIV. Respite unit,
information and support centre,
buddy programme and
women's weekly support group.

LOSS AND BEREAVEMENT

The Compassionate Friends

53 North Street
Bristol BS3 1EN
Helpline: 0845 123 2304
Tel: 0845 120 3785
Email: info@tcf.org.uk
www.tcf.org.uk

Nationwide organisation of, and
for, bereaved parents offering
friendship and understanding
to other bereaved parents.

CRUSE – Bereavement Care Scotland

Riverview House (Headquarters)
Friarton Road
Perth PH2 8DF
Tel: 01738 444 178
Email: info@crusescotland.org.uk
www.crusescotland.org.uk

Help, support and counselling
for bereaved people.

Foundation for the Study of Infant Deaths (FSID)

Artillery House
11–19 Artillery Row
London SW1P 1RT
Tel: 020 7222 8001
Helpline: 020 7233 2090 (24 hour)
Email: office@fsid.org.uk
www.fsid.org.uk

Personal support and information
for parents who have lost a child
through cot death. Runs the Care
of Next Infant (CONI) programme,
providing support and advice for
families bereaved by cot death
with subsequent children.

Scottish Cot Death Trust

Royal Hospital for Sick Children
Yorkhill
Glasgow G3 8SJ
Tel: 0141 357 3946
Email: contact@sidsscotland.org.uk
www.sidscotland.org.uk

Support and information for
parents bereaved by sudden
infant death. Puts parents in
touch with local support groups
or other bereaved parents.

Stillbirth and Neonatal Death Society (SANDS)

28 Portland Place
London W1B 1LY
Helpline: 020 7436 5881 (weekdays)
Email: support@uk-sands.org
www.uk-sands.org

Information and a national
network of support groups
for bereaved parents.

MENTAL HEALTH

Association for Postnatal Illness (APNI)

145 Dawes Road
Fulham
London SW6 7EB
Tel: 020 7386 0868
Email: info@apni.org
www.apni.org

A network of telephone and
postal volunteers who have
suffered from postnatal illness
and offer information, support
and encouragement on a
one-to-one basis.

Meet A Mum Association (MAMA)

54 Lillington Road
Radstock BA3 3NR
Tel: 0845 120 6162 (Mon–Fri 7–10 pm)
Helpline: 0845 120 3746
Email: meet_a_mum.assoc@
btinternet.com
www.mama.co.uk

Helps mothers and mothers-to-be
who are isolated and lonely by
putting them in touch with others
for friendship and support.

The Samaritans

Helpline: 08457 90 90 90
Email: jo@samaritans.org
www.samaritans.org

Provides confidential, non-
judgemental support, 24 hours a
day for people experiencing feelings
of distress or despair, including those
which could lead to suicide.

Scottish Association for Mental Health (SAMH)

Cumbrae House
15 Carlton Court
Glasgow G5 9JP
Tel: 0141 568 7000
Email: enquire@samh.org.uk
www.samh.org.uk

Offers an information service,
campaigning, and training on
mental health issues. Deals
with any queries on the subject
of mental health, and legal and,
or benefits services.

Young Minds

48–50 Saint John Street
London EC1M 4DG
Tel: 020 7336 8445
Parents Information Service:
0800 018 2138
Email: enquiries@youngminds.org.uk
www.youngminds.org.uk

A national charity committed to
improving the mental health of all
children and young people under 25.

ORAL HEALTH

Childsmile

Cameron House
Cameron Bridge
Leven
Fife KY8 5RG
Tel: 01592 226 416
www.child-smile.org

An early years tooth decay
prevention programme. Provides
information on nursery and
school programmes and
promotes oral health from birth.

PARENT SUPPORT

Bliss

2nd Floor, 9 Holyrood Street
London Bridge
London SE1 2EL
Parent Support Helpline:
0500 618 140
Tel: 020 7378 1122
Email: information@bliss.org.uk
www.bliss.org.uk

Provides education, resources
and support for parents and carers
of babies who are, or have been,
in special care.

Bookbug Programme

Scottish Book Trust
Sandeman House
55 Trunk's Close
Edinburgh
EH1 1SR
Tel: 0131 524 0180
Email: bookbug@scottishbooktrust.
com
www.scottishbooktrust.com

A national programme that
encourages parents to share and
enjoy books with their children.

Contact a family

Helpline: 0808 808 3555
(10 am–4.00 pm and
5.30 pm–7.30 pm,
Monday to Friday)
www.cafamily.org.uk

A charity providing support,
advice and information for
families with disabled children.

Cry-sis

BM CRY-sis
London WC1N 3XX
Helpline: 08451 228 669
Email: info@cry-sis.org.uk
www.cry-sis.org.uk

Self-help and support for families
with excessively crying, sleepless
and demanding children via
national helpline. Also by
post – please enclose SAE.

Gingerbread Scotland

1014 Argyle Street
Glasgow G3 8TD
Tel: 0141 286 1595
Helpline: 0808 802 0925
(9 am–5 pm Mondays to Friday,
9 am–8 pm Wednesday)

Local groups offer mutual support,
friendship, information, advice
and practical help to one-parent
families. Welcomes pregnant women.

Home-Start

2 Salisbury Road
Leicester LE1 7QR
Information Line: 0800 068 6368
Tel: 0116 233 9955
Email: info@home-start.org.uk
www.home-start.org.uk

Offers friendly, practical help
and emotional support to families
who may be experiencing stress
(must have at least one child
under five years old).

One Parent Families Scotland

13 Gayfield Square
Edinburgh EH1 3NX
Helpline: 0808 801 0323
Tel: 0131 556 3899
Email: info@opfs.org.uk
www.opfs.org.uk

The national voluntary organisation
for lone parents offering family
support services and a range
of help and information.

Play Talk Read
www.infoscotland.com/playtalkread

A website with a wealth of ideas,
activities and materials to get you
playing, talking and reading with
your baby.

Tommy's

Nicholas House
3 Laurence Pountney Hill
London EC4R 0BB
Tel: 020 7398 3483 (pregnancy
information line)
Email: info@tommys.org
www.tommys.org/pregnancy

Information and advice on having
a healthy pregnancy to women
and their partners. You can also
order free books and leaflets from
the website, including 'The young
woman's guide to pregnancy', which
is aimed at women aged 16–19.

Twins and Multiple Births Association (TAMBA)

2 The Willows
Gardner Road
Guildford
Surrey GU1 4PJ
Tel: 01483 304 442
Helpline: 0800 138 0509 (evenings)
Email: enquiries@tamba.org.uk
www.tamba.org.uk

Aims to provide information and mutual support networks for families of twins, triplets and more, highlighting their unique needs to all involved in their care.

Fatherhood Institute

9 Nevill Street
Abergavenny NP7 5AA
Tel: 0845 634 1328
Email: mail@fatherhoodinstitute.org
www.fathersdirect.com

A UK-wide information centre for fathers. The website has a special section for new dads.

Parentline Scotland

Tel: 0808 800 2222
www.children1st.org.uk/parentline

A telephone helpline service which gives parents the chance to ask about things that are worrying them and points them to useful services or information.

Parenting Across Scotland

c/o Children 1st
1 Boroughloch Square
Edinburgh EH8 9NJ
Tel: 0131 319 8060
Email: alison.clancy@children1st.org.uk
www.parentingacrossscotland.org

A partnership of relationship organisations and children's charities working together on issues affecting parents and families in Scotland today.

PREGNANCY AND MATERNITY SERVICES

AIMS (Association for Improvements in the Maternity Service)

40 Leamington Terrace
Edinburgh EH10 4JL
Tel: 0870 765 1451
Helpline: 0870 765 1433
Email: secretary@aims.org.uk
www.aims.org.uk

A voluntary pressure group offering support and information about parents' rights, complaints procedures and choices within maternity care, including home birth.

Birth Resource Centre Edinburgh

18 Saint Peters Place
Viewforth
Edinburgh EH3 9PH
Tel: 0131 229 3667
Email: info@birthresourcecentre.org.uk
www.pregnancyandparents.org.uk

Practical and emotional support for all women and their families: antenatal and postnatal classes, one-to-one support, sharing experiences, information, advocacy and child-centred activities.

Doula UK

PO Box 26678
London N14 4WB
Tel: 01438 236 510
www.doula.org.uk

A network which offers advice on finding a doula in your area.

PREGNANCY PROBLEMS

Action on Pre-eclampsia (APEC)

2c The Halfcroft
Syston LE7 1LD
Helpline: 020 8427 4217
Email: info@apec.org.uk
www.apec.org.uk

Charity providing support and information for sufferers of pre-eclampsia.

Antenatal Results and Choices (ARC)

73 Charlotte Street
London W1T 4PN
Helpline: 020 7631 0285
Email: info@arc-uk.org
www.arc-uk.org

Offers support and information to women and couples who have had a diagnosis of abnormality in their unborn baby, and provides continued support to those parents who have a termination of pregnancy.

The Chartered Association of Physiotherapy

14 Bedford Row
London WC1R 4ED
Tel: 020 7306 6666
Email: enquiries@csp.org.uk
www.csp.org.uk

Information regarding the role and function of a chartered physiotherapist, including how to get in touch with local private practitioners.

Miscarriage Association

c/o Clayton Hospital
Northgate
Wakefield WF1 3JS
West Yorkshire
Scottish Helpline: 0131 334 8883
Email: info@miscarriageassociation.org.uk
www.miscarriageassociation.org.uk

Information, advice and support for women suffering the effects of miscarriage.

SCIM (Scottish Care and Information on Miscarriage)

285 High Street
Glasgow G4 0QS
Tel: 0141 552 5070
www.miscarriagesupport.org.uk
Email: miscarriagescotland@hotmail.com

A counselling service for women who have lost babies through miscarriage, offering support for future pregnancy and planning pregnancy following loss.

Pelvic Instability Network Scotland (PINS)

Suilven
Southend
Argyll PA28 6RF
Email: info@pelvicinstability.org.uk
www.pelvicinstability.org.uk

Registered Scottish charity providing support and information to people affected by pelvic girdle pain.

RIGHTS AND BENEFITS

ACAS (Advisory, Conciliation and Arbitration Service)

151 West George Street
Glasgow G2 7JJ
Tel: 0141 248 1400
Minicom: 0845 606 1600
Helpline: 0845 747 4747
www.acas.org.uk

Provides advice on time-off for antenatal care and on matters such as unfair dismissal.

Benefit Enquiry Line

0800 88 22 00
Textphone: 0800 24 33 55

A confidential telephone advice and information service for people with disabilities, their carers and representatives. Offers general advice and information about social security benefits and how to claim them.

Child Benefit Office

PO Box 1
Newcastle Upon Tyne NE88 1AA
Tel: 0845 302 1444
Textphone: 0845 302 1474
Email: child.benefit@ir.gsi.gov.uk
www.inlandrevenue.gov.uk/childbenefit/

Offers advice and information about Child Benefits, One Parent Benefit and Guardian's Allowance.

Child Support Agency

PO Box 55
Brierly Hill
West Midlands DY5 1YL
Tel: 08457 133 133
Textphone: 08457 138 924
www.csa.gov.uk

The government agency that assesses and collects child maintenance in Great Britain.

Citizens Advice Bureaux (CABs)

Ask at your local library or look in your phone book under 'Counselling and Advice' or 'Citizens Advice Bureau'.

Equality and Human Rights Commission

The Optima Building
58 Robertson Street
Glasgow G2 8DU
Tel: 0845 604 5510
Email: Scotlandhelpline@equalityhumanrights.com

Information and advice on issues of discrimination and equal opportunities.

Edinburgh Disability Benefits Centre

PO Box 38
Edinburgh EH91 5AJ

Information and advice on Attendance Allowance and Disability Living Allowance.

Glasgow Disability Benefits Centre

PO Box 37
Glasgow G90 8AS
Tel: 0141 249 3500
Email: glasgowdbc/customerservice@dwp.gsi.gov.uk

Information and advice on Attendance Allowance and Disability Living Allowance.

Jobcentre Plus (Department of Work and Pensions)

www.jobcentreplus.gov.uk

For general advice on all social security benefits, child support, pensions and National Insurance, including maternity benefits and income support. Telephone, write or call in to Jobcentre Plus – look up Jobcentre Plus in the phone book for local details.

Parent's guide to money

www.moneymadeclear.org.uk/parents/home.html

Social Services and Welfare Organisations

For information on topics including benefits, housing, financial difficulties, employment, relationship problems, childcare and useful organisations. Look up the entry in the phone book under the name of your local authority or ask at your local library or Citizen's Advice Bureau.

Scottish Refugee Council

5 Cadogan Square
Glasgow G2 7PH
Tel: 0141 2489 799
Email: info@scottishrefugeecouncil.org.uk
www.scottishrefugeecouncil.org.uk

Freephone number for newly arrived and dispersed asylum seekers: 0800 085 6087
(9.30 am–4.30 pm Monday to Friday)

VEGETARIANISM

Vegetarian Society of the UK Ltd

Parkdale
Dunham Road
Altrincham
Cheshire WA14 4QG
Tel: 0161 925 2000
Email: info@vegsoc.org
www.vegsoc.org

For general information and advice on all aspects of vegetarianism.

Glossary

Most groups of people have their jargon, and health professionals are no exception. Here's a list of some common words or acronyms (initials) or abbreviations which you may come across when you read your notes or hear people talking. If in doubt, ask your midwife or doctor what they mean.

AFP: alphafetoprotein. A substance present in the blood of pregnant women. You may need further tests if your levels appear higher or lower than normal.

ALB: albumin. This is a protein. If it's present in your urine, it may be a sign of pre-eclampsia or of an infection such as cystitis.

AMNIOTIC FLUID: sometimes called liquor (pronounced lye-kwor), this is the fluid that surrounds the baby in the uterus.

ANTENATAL: before the birth.

APH: stands for antepartum haemorrhage and means bleeding before the birth.

BR: breech presentation. A baby who is lying bottom or feet down in the uterus.

BP: blood pressure. It's important to have your blood pressure measured as a rise could mean a problem.

CEPH: cephalic. Presentation of the baby with her head in the lower part of the uterus.

ECTOPIC PREGNANCY: a pregnancy that develops somewhere other than the uterus, usually in the fallopian tube. This pregnancy cannot be allowed to continue as it is dangerous.

EDD: expected date of delivery – when your baby is due. Sometimes called EDC (expected date of confinement).

ENG: engaged. Means that the widest diameter of the baby's head has passed into the pelvis in preparation for giving birth.

EPISIOTOMY: a cut made in the mother's perineum (the area between the vagina and anus) to allow the baby to be born more quickly and prevent tearing.

FETUS: medical name for the baby before it's born.

FH: fetal heart. You may see 'FH heard' or 'FHH' on your notes – that means your baby's heartbeat has been heard.

FM: fetal movement. It may say 'FM felt' or 'FMF' on your notes. That means your baby has been felt to move.

FUNDUS: this is the top of the uterus. The 'fundal height' helps assess the growth of the baby and how many weeks pregnant you are. It's the length in centimetres between the top of the uterus and the pubic bone.

Hb: haemoglobin. This gives an indication of iron levels in your blood. If it's too low, it could mean you have anaemia and need more iron.

HYPERTENSION: high blood pressure.

HYPOTENSION: low blood pressure.

LMP: last menstrual period. This date is used to work out how many weeks pregnant you are.

MULTIGRAVIDA: a woman who has been pregnant before.

MULTIPARA: also called multip – a woman who has given birth at least once before.

NAD: nothing abnormal detected. The doctor or midwife may write this on your notes when they find no problems.

OCCIPITO ANTERIOR: means the back of your baby's head is towards your front. You may see LOA or ROA on your notes which means left (or right) occipito anterior and describes whether the baby's head is towards the left or the right. LOA is usually the best position for a shorter labour and an easier birth.

OCCIPITO POSTERIOR: as above but the baby's head is towards your back.

OEDEMA: means swelling. Fluid retention can cause swelling in your ankles, fingers and elsewhere. You may see it measured in your notes as + or ++.

PALPATION: when the midwife or doctor feels the baby by moving their hands across your abdomen.

PERINEUM: the area of skin between your vagina and anus.

PIH: pregnancy-induced hypertension. Means that your blood pressure is high.

PLACENTA PRAEVIA: when the placenta is low down. Sometimes it covers the cervix and blocks the baby's exit, which could mean you need a Caesarean section.

POSITION: how the baby is lying, for example to the right or left of the pelvis.

POSTNATAL: after the birth.

PRESENTATION: the part of the baby which is coming first (usually the crown or back of the baby's head).

PRETERM: born before 37 weeks of pregnancy.

PRIMIGRAVIDA: a woman pregnant for the first time.

PRIMIPARA: sometimes called prim or primip – a woman giving birth for the first time.

QUICKENING: the first movements of the baby that you can feel.

Rh: rhesus. The rhesus blood group system is a way of categorising your blood type.

ROOMING IN: most maternity units now recommend that babies stay with their mums 24 hours a day. This helps with feeding and bonding. It also reduces the risk of infection.

SKIN-TO-SKIN: skin-to-skin contact with your baby after birth (your baby is dried and put straight onto your chest).

SYNTOCINON: drug given during third stage of labour to assist with delivery of placenta.

TERM: 40 weeks or thereabouts from the first day of the last menstrual period.

VE: vaginal examination.

VENTOUSE: vacuum extractions. Sometimes used to help the baby out.

VX: stands for vertex, which means the crown or top of the baby's head.

Index

A

absent-mindedness, 51

abuse,
    child, 197
    domestic, 30, 197

acceleration of labour, 70
    see also induction

accident prevention
and safety, 197

actively managed
delivery of placenta, 70, 104

acupressure, 73

acupuncture, 73

adoption, 197

advice,
    for new mums, 113
    on breastfeeding, 57–8
    on crying, 142
    on postnatal depression,
    113, 158–63
    unasked for, 49

aerobics (low-impact), 8
    see also exercise

AFP (alphafetoprotein), 208

AIDS (acquired immune
deficiency syndrome), 37, 203

airbags and car seats,
83, 133, 187

ALB (albumin), 208

albumin, 208

alcohol,
    during breastfeeding, 12, 124
    during pregnancy, 12, 21
    helpful addresses, 197

allergies, *see* peanuts
    feeding and, 174
    weaning and, 172

amniocentesis, 32, 39, 41

amniotic fluid, 54, 208

anaemia, 50

anaesthesia (epidural), 73, 80
    see also Caesarean section

anaphylaxis, 199

anencephaly, 40

animals (contact with), 19
    and hand washing, 139

ankles (swollen), 48, 65, 67, 69
    see also oedema

antenatal care, 4, 24
    booking appointment, 25
    classes, 44–5, 53
    diagnostic tests, 39
    routine checks, 38
    routine tests, 36–7
    staff involved in, 28–9

antenatal classes, 44–5
    sharing worries at, 53

antenatal notes, 27

antenatal rights, 35
    see also maternity leave

antibodies in
breast milk, 122–5

Apgar score, 101, 105

APH (antepartum
haemorrhage), 208

appetite
    of baby, 120
    of mother, 47

aquanatal classes, 9

asking for help, 113, 149, 205

assisting birth, 100

asthma, 122, 200

attachment for feeding, 127

autism, 201

B

baby (born),
    adequate feeding, 121
    appearance at birth, 101
    bathing, 134–7
    clothes for, 140
    crying, 142
    development,

        first days, 111
        1–2 months, 154–5
        3–4 months, 164–5
        5–6 months, 168–9
        7–8 months, 180–1
        9–10 months, 182–3
        11–12 months, 188–9
    equipment for, 141
    first 24 hours, 106
    foods for weaning 172–7
    getting to know, 102, 110
    see also bonding
    immunisation of, 156–7
    position for sleeping, 144
    routine care,
        bathing, 134–7
        nappies, 138–40
    routine testing, 114–16
    special care, 117
    teething, 178–9
    the sleepy/reluctant
    feeder, 127
    weaning, 172–7

baby (unborn), *see* fetus

baby blues, 113
    see also postnatal depression

baby massage, 143

baby slings, 141

baby-led (demand) feeding, 122

babysitting, 171

back carriers, 141

backache, 47–8, 58, 78

bacteria, food preparation
and, 19, 20

bathing, 134–5
    drowning, 187
    step-by-step, 136–7

bearing down, 98

bed sharing, 145

behavioural difficulties, 198

benefits,
    Child Benefit, 64
    Child Trust Fund, 64